IT'S ALL IN YOUR BODY

Dr Sula Windgassen

IT'S ALL IN YOUR BODY

A Practical Roadmap to Healing
Through Mind–Body Connection

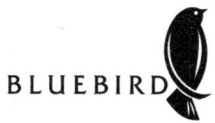

First published 2026 by Bluebird
an imprint of Pan Macmillan
The Smithson, 6 Briset Street, London EC1M 5NR
EU representative: Macmillan Publishers Ireland Ltd, 1st Floor,
The Liffey Trust Centre, 117–126 Sheriff Street Upper,
Dublin 1 D01 YC43
Associated companies throughout the world

HB ISBN 978-1-0350-5814-3
TPB ISBN 978-1-0350-5815-0

Copyright © Sula Windgassen 2026

The right of Sula Windgassen to be identified as the
author of this work has been asserted in accordance with
the Copyright, Designs and Patents Act 1988.

All rights reserved. No part of this publication may be reproduced, stored in
a retrieval system, or transmitted, in any form, or by any means (including,
without limitation, electronic, mechanical, photocopying, recording or
otherwise) without the prior written permission of the publisher.

Pan Macmillan does not have any control over, or any responsibility for,
any author or third-party websites (including, without limitation, URLs,
emails and QR codes) referred to in or on this book.

1 3 5 7 9 8 6 4 2

A CIP catalogue record for this book is available from the British Library.

Typeset in Kepler Std by Six Red Marbles UK, Thetford, Norfolk
Printed and bound in the UK using 100% Renewable Electricity by CPI Group (UK) Ltd

This book contains the opinions and ideas of its author. It is intended to provide helpful general
information on the subjects that it addresses. It is not in any way a substitute for the advice of the
reader's own physician(s) or other medical professionals based on the reader's own individual
conditions, symptoms, or concerns. If the reader needs personal medical, health, dietary, exercise,
or other assistance or advice, the reader should consult a competent physician and/ or other
qualified health care professionals. The author and publisher specifically disclaim all responsibility
for injury, damage, or loss that the reader may incur as a direct or indirect consequence of following
any directions or suggestions given in the book or participating in any programs described in the
book. The reader is advised not to undertake, cease, or modify any treatments, diets, or health
procedures without consulting a professional. Failure to adhere to this recommendation may result
in adverse health impacts, for which the author and publisher accept no responsibility.

This book is sold subject to the condition that it shall not, by way of trade or otherwise,
be lent, hired out, or otherwise circulated without the publisher's prior consent in any
form of binding or cover other than that in which it is published and without a similar condition
including this condition being imposed on the subsequent purchaser. The publisher does not
authorize the use or reproduction of any part of this book in any manner for the purpose of
training artificial intelligence technologies or systems. The publisher expressly reserves
this book from the Text and Data Mining exception in accordance with Article 4(3) of the
European Union Digital Single Market Directive 2019/790.

Visit **www.panmacmillan.com/bluebird** to read more about
all our books and to buy them.

For those who have felt unseen in your suffering. May you come to know yourself with wisdom and compassion.

CONTENTS

Preface ix

Introduction: All in your head or all in your body? 1

SECTION ONE: Understanding your body 33

Chapter 1: Befriending your biology 37
Chapter 2: Mind–body interactions 69

SECTION TWO: Transforming your experience of symptoms 103

Chapter 3: Interrupting symptom spirals 107
Chapter 4: Biology balancing behaviour 133
Chapter 5: Feeling yourself better 167
Chapter 6: Thinking yourself better or thinking yourself sick? 193
Chapter 7: It's not all on you 225

SECTION THREE: Sustaining change and becoming who you are 269

Chapter 8: Updating your beliefs 273
Chapter 9: A beautiful work in progress 303

Acknowledgements 329
Index 331
Link to Notes 349

PREFACE

You may be one of the people who experiences everyday life with a difference. Pushing a full supermarket trolley down an aisle and grimacing as the effort flares up your pain. Running for the bus and suddenly stopping short, dropping your head between your legs with a dizziness that threatens to cut the day short. Sat at home drafting messages to cancel plans that should be exciting but instead feel scary. Perhaps from a young age your health or mood has required extra consideration and navigation. Or maybe for a long time, you had an idea of what the future held until things changed. Mystery symptoms, unexpected diagnoses or complications from routine procedures – life can blindside you. Some life twists have nothing to do with physical health, coming instead from traumas, relationship breakdowns, job losses and bereavements. They might have nothing to do with physical health, until they do. Whatever your specific situation, grappling with physical symptoms, ill-health or mood difficulties can be a huge challenge and make you question your sense of self. I know because I've been there.

I wrote this book for anyone experiencing physical and emotional challenges, so that you can move from feeling attacked by your own mind and body to feeling empowered to work with them. This book will help if you feel stuck in spirals of overthinking, overwhelm and hopelessness that are by now all too familiar, but seem impossible to change. From IBS to burnout, bladder issues to multiple mystery symptoms, cancer recovery to endometriosis, this is a book for those who are fed up of feeling alone in project-managing their own health and wellbeing.

Whether you have a chronic illness/disability, support those who do, or feel sabotaged by your own brain, this book provides a holistic way to work with your biology to reconnect with yourself and to feel better physically and emotionally. In this book, you will find a non-judgemental guide to help you understand symptom patterns in a way that you have probably not encountered before, so that you can be empowered to transform your experience. You'll set your own healing goals and navigate your way towards them by learning about the mysteries of mind–body communication, how to change this communication and how to better meet your own needs with practical strategies. As you move through the sections of this book, you will come to connect with your own unconditional worth, present in sickness and in health.

I am a health psychologist who focusses on improving health through the use of psychology, and this book is the culmination of years of study, research and clinical practice. My professional endeavours, however, were driven by my own personal health experiences which turned my life upside down, making me question how I could ever be OK again. To illustrate the science, I have pulled from my own experience of remission from bladder issues and my clinical work with patients. For transparency and reliability, I have cited primary research sources, using where possible the highest quality published research, such as systematic reviews and meta-analyses.[*] To preserve the privacy, trust and wellbeing of the people I have worked with, I have used a process adopted by clinical academics for lecturing, so that all identifiable details have been abstracted and anonymized. Depictions of therapeutic changes and outcomes will be accurate when described.

In this book, there may be case studies that sound exactly like you, or someone you know. My work has shown me just how much

---

[*] A collation of the results of high-quality studies on a given topic.

commonality there is across people's experiences of illness, burnout and trauma, and yet so many face these challenges alone. This can lead you to conclude that there is something wrong with you; you're not strong enough, capable enough, cared for enough. And yet my work and research shows that this is not a '*you* problem' at all. Hopefully, seeing instances of your own experience in the stories of others can help to reassure you of that.

How do you feel as you begin this book? Perhaps things are bleak and you feel sceptical. Maybe you feel an urgency, anxiously hoping *this* is the answer. My wish for you is that this book opens new avenues of hope, while calming the desperate need for certainty. That where there were once dead ends, blame and stigma, there will be choices, empowering experiences and a growing self-compassion. That knowing you will be OK is no longer based on precarious signs or the unreliability of others, but from a growing wisdom that comes from uniting mind and body.

INTRODUCTION

All in your head or all in your body?

'It's all in your head' is a phrase you may be familiar with. It's a sentiment often communicated implicitly and explicitly in healthcare systems and society when there are not clear answers or solutions for complex issues. I believe it is a harmful message that inhibits healing. As a health psychologist, who uses psychology to improve physical health, I have seen first-hand the incredible ways that psychology can physically shift biological processes in the body, but this doesn't mean your symptoms are 'in your head'. As we begin this journey together, I'll introduce you to an alternative way of using psychology to improve health, working with your biology, as we begin to set healing goals to instil hope. But first, I'd like to share my story of a mystery illness in my twenties that drastically changed my life.

I was working as a marketing manager, having recently finished my psychology degree, when I started to get back-to-back urinary tract infections. Up until this point, I had had fleeting and repeating infections since childhood that cleared up with antibiotics or cystitis sachets. Not this time though. Having never experienced complete symptom remission, what had once been an irritating inconvenience quickly became disconcerting. Going to pee was something I had to brace myself for, not knowing if it would result in the most intense and painful urge to wee without the ability to actually pass anything. I'd writhe in agony, with the urgent feeling I was about to wet myself, without ever reaching the relief of passing water. Imagine needing the toilet so badly you can't hold it in any longer. You run to the bathroom and nothing comes out. But this feeling of urgency only gets more intense. And now it burns. The burning radiates up your urethra, to your stomach. And now, you feel physically sick. This was my every day and it caused me a deep sense of dread every time I needed to go to the toilet.

After months of this, the migraines came. They would arrive in the middle of the night, violently ripping me from sleep, as sharp throbbing from my temple radiated across my skull, my eyes watering yet squeezed tightly shut under the immense pressure. The migraines were so painful I initially reacted by banging my head against the wall – not something I'd recommend. Sleep was my only escape from these migraines and yet it was near impossible to sleep because of the pain, leaving me tossing and turning in agony until the early hours. No painkillers worked and I couldn't find any other solutions, which left me in a terrified stalemate bracing for the next uncontrollable attack.

These symptoms and more, combined with the side effects of the multiple medications I was already taking, meant that I had to be signed off work. It had been about six months and the overwhelming stress of having these symptoms was wearing me down physically and mentally. I didn't have the capacity to figure out how to change things by myself. As a recent psychology graduate and daughter of a psychiatrist, I sought the help of a therapist.

I wanted them to help me learn to work with my body when it was making me feel so bad. I wanted someone who could give me practical advice to navigate the difficult decisions I was having to make. Someone who could help me feel less ashamed of myself and my sense of worthlessness. Unfortunately, I got none of those things.

It was a Friday evening, already dark, and my dad was driving me back to Leeds to my first therapy appointment. I had moved back home with him, hoping to rehabilitate my ailing body. I was having migraines every other day, rather than daily, with a semblance of hope that maybe the pain would go and that my bladder might calm down. *Then* I could resume life. After therapy I would be going back to my apartment to try and regain some independence.

We left the motorway, now on the familiar stretch that brought me into the city that had been my home for years. My head began to throb. I was unsure if the sick feeling in my stomach was anxiety that a migraine might begin or the migraine beginning. My dad and I looked at each other, agreeing it likely was no coincidence that the pain had struck at this very moment. I considered cancelling my therapy appointment, but at such short notice it would be chargeable, and I figured that I was bound to have multiple migraines during the therapy sessions ahead as they were so relentless.

In that first session, my therapist assessed me, as I pressed a cold bottle to my right temple, head bent to one side, legs curled up and coat still on. I explained I was in a lot of pain but as I was always in pain there had been no point cancelling. This was barely acknowledged. I explained why I had come to therapy. That I knew my panic about my symptoms was making them worse, but that it was hard not to panic when the symptoms were so scary. None of this was explored.

There were a lot of questions about my childhood, and I was wary that there weren't many questions about my health. But in good faith, I decided to show up to subsequent appointments, hoping they would start to give me some direction. I *needed* help. It was after my third appointment that I decided I would not go back to therapy. During this appointment I told my therapist that my bladder symptoms had flared up after my boyfriend and I had sex. Sex and cystitis are unfortunately not uncommon bedfellows, particularly if you are prone to bladder infections. This is not news to a lot of people, less so to women, even less so to GPs and much less so to urologists. I flippantly shared that I hadn't bothered telling the urologist that I'd flared up *because* of sex, because my dad was in the consultation and it would have been a bit awkward. It was at this moment that the therapist said to me, 'So even though you were in pain, having these *awful* symptoms' – this was the first time, by the way, that he'd acknowledged how awful the symptoms were – 'you did not tell your doctor because you were *ashamed* to talk about sex in front of your dad?'

He paused, as though he had said something meaningful. In my attempts to clarify my situation, the reality of my condition, and that what I really wanted his help with right now was a decision about whether or not to get my urethra stretched, it felt like I had not spoken at all. Like a dream where you try to talk but the words are stuck. He could not hear me, no matter how clear I was, and it felt terrifying. *Why could no one understand that I was freaking out about my body doing all these things that physically hurt me and that I had no control over?*

If you have health issues, you may be familiar with the spirals that ensued. *Was I just overreacting? Was I making my symptoms worse than they were?* Mixed with the fear, came the loathing. *Maybe I was just a little, pathetic weakling.*

The loathing gave way to anger. *Why were people not helping me? Why couldn't they answer my questions when I had been as clear as I could be?*

And this gave way to fear and despair again. *Maybe this therapist and everyone else like him weren't answering my questions because they couldn't. Maybe I was truly on my own to figure it all out.* And *that* felt impossible.

This experience of therapy (my first) came the best part of a year after my symptoms had started, having shapeshifted and intensified into a whole range of other symptoms. Before starting therapy, I had tirelessly searched for solutions and seen all the GPs in my surgery and then my dad's. I even remember a lovely GP close to retiring, who took me to his car boot to give me some numbing gel to see if that would work, at a loss for anything else to suggest. I had been to gynaecologists, urologists, and had tried multiple treatments. Many of which came with horrible side effects, without any benefit.

I'd grown ever more hopeless, depressed and even suicidal. I couldn't fathom the point of living if it was going to be so painful. I had taken unpaid sick leave and moved back in with my dad temporarily. Serendipitously, my dad was doing a master's degree in mindfulness at the time and his partner worked as a psychologist in a pain clinic. They educated me on pain processes and what was happening in my brain and nervous system when I got these infections, and how a practice like mindfulness could change things. When I sought therapy, I was hoping the therapist would help me better understand this and guide me in practices to calm my frazzled nervous system to improve my physical and mental health.

I felt too vulnerable when I ended therapy to find another therapist. Instead, I threw myself into mindfulness and embodiment practices that helped cultivate safety in my body. The more I practised, the less alarmed I felt by symptoms and the more they seemed to change for the better. Months on, there was no pain any more and the migraines were gone. I still felt bladder discomfort and I needed to go to the toilet very frequently, but it was no longer an event that terrified me.

I got a pet rabbit (relevant mainly because he really soothed and amused me, which you'll come to appreciate in its significance for positively shifting biological processes later) and made plans to leave the job I now hated to make the move from Leeds to London to study for a master's in health psychology at the prestigious Institute of Psychiatry, Psychology and Neuroscience at King's College London. I had a mission. I wanted to understand the processes of the mind–body connection so that I could do two things: a) get rid of my overactive bladder, and b) improve the experiences of other people with different physiology and psychology to me.

In the year I moved to London to study for my master's, I went for more invasive diagnostic tests (without any definitive answers), got obsessively into 'clean eating' and supplementation and tried every naturopathic supplement under the sun. The master's course was intense. I was managing health appointments, working two jobs and doing my full-time master's degree with a placement and research dissertation, while trying to stay afloat in the London economy. I still felt acutely aware of my bladder and during that year there were periods where it really affected me, as I will share with you later in the book.

They say healing isn't linear. And it really is not. I continued to practise mindfulness, incorporated strategies from cognitive behavioural therapy I was learning about and scaled back my frenzied micromanagement of my body through rigid health regimes. Meanwhile, other things were fundamentally changing. I had found meaning and purpose again. And this was connecting me with others who shared the same interests and passions, who made me feel seen and understood. The more I felt aligned with my purpose and the more I felt a sense of belonging, the less urgency I had to fix each niggling symptom. And over the course of the year, I was symptom free.

I was inspired by the patients I met on my placement and in conducting my thesis (an exploration of the effect of mindfulness in progressive multiple sclerosis) and I felt galvanized to better understand all of these processes on behalf of them and others who may never be able to get symptom remission. This journey was no longer about me. I was traumatized by the depths of despair and pain I had felt, and I couldn't bear the idea that others would be trapped in similar or worse experiences. So, when the opportunity came to deepen my understanding and study for a PhD exploring how psychological therapy could physically create changes in gut symptoms, I jumped at the opportunity. Well, almost – I had a minor freak-out about finances and then resolved that I would make it work.

Over the following four years I completed two doctoral qualifications, publishing over twenty scientific papers on the topic of mind–body interventions, some of which made national headlines because of how effective the interventions were at physically improving symptoms.[1] I worked on trials exploring the use of psychology in irritable bowel syndrome, inflammatory bowel disease,[2] and multiple sclerosis,[3] collating definitive themes of how mind–body miscommunication was occurring and how it could be improved for better physical and mental health.

I consider myself to be lucky in my journey because it was not strategic. I was fortunate to have fundamental information shared, experiences that made me curious and a support network that facilitated my explorations and healing. My academic work helped me to make retrospective sense of what changed my physiology, pulling out the pieces of the puzzle coherently.

The relationship between physical health and psychology now much clearer, I knew I had to deepen my understanding of mental-health processes. I had seen how the lack of integration between mental and physical healthcare systems left people stuck between services. I applied for a funded place to train as a psychotherapist in the National Health Service (NHS), starting a new phase of my journey to support others with mental and physical health issues.

Years later, working as a therapist on the long-term condition pathway in the NHS, it was my job to provide specialized therapy for people with chronic health issues. Sat in a fraying but plump mint-green armchair, clipboard in lap, tapestries of sunlight dancing across the whiteboard, I'd see the full spectrum of expressions reflecting the same fear: blank and shut-down faces, eyes darting around, trying to make sense of what was happening, cheeks red with anger. And then there were the glistening eyes that pleaded, 'Please take me seriously.' It would sometimes take the full course of therapy for them to trust that I wasn't simply telling them to 'stress less'.

This work made me realize that societally, in our medical systems and collective responses to health issues, we are not *really* familiar with how mind (psychology) and body (biology/physiology) interact. This lack of familiarity gives rise to stigmatizing assumptions, such as: if psychology influences your physical health, then it a) caused your health issues to begin with, and b) is your fault and up to you alone to control and improve things.

This is why I wanted to write this book. To make the use of psychology for improving health less stigmatizing and more effective. This work involves updating your understanding of the relationship between your biology and your psychology. Rather than one causing the other, the two are intertwined. Every human experience is biologically mediated. By this I mean, you wouldn't be able to have a thought, to feel an emotion or to react without the biological processes happening within you (e.g. brain activity, breathing, hormonal shifts and neurochemical transmissions, etc.). The conversation between psychology and biology is continuous. This conversation can escalate into an argument, with mind protesting the body and vice versa.

Have you ever tried to work but your mind keeps going off track? This is an example of a mind–body stand-off. As is feeling angry at your body for being sick. These stand-offs can derail mind–body communication with the effect of physically worsening symptoms and mental health. To physically improve symptoms and mental health, the mind–body communication needs to be harmonious and collaborative.

My research and clinical practice with hundreds of patients, led me to create a 'biopsychosocial' psychotherapeutic framework that helps bridge the gap between physiology and psychology. This approach is distinct from traditional models of psychotherapy, that purely target mental health as a means of improving physical health. Figure 1 illustrates the distinction, which becomes particularly important when people, depleted by health issues and seeking support, are made to feel that their mental health is the issue, not the other way round. Or where improving mental health is portrayed as simply thinking better. The biopsychosocial

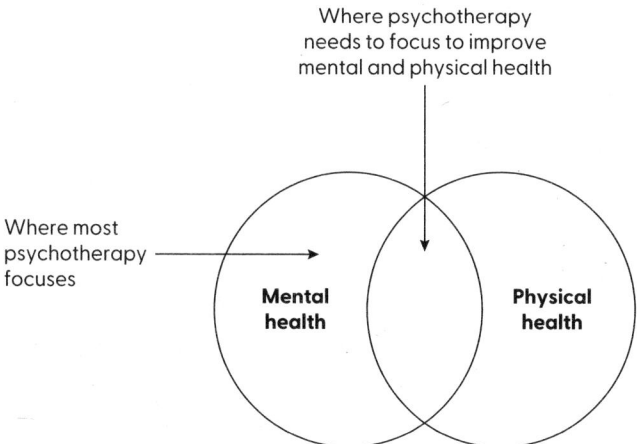

Figure 1: Where traditional mental health models of psychotherapy focus compared to where the biopsychosocial psychotherapeutic framework focusses: the interplay between psychology and biology (mental health and physical health).

psychotherapeutic framework is one I use in my clinical practice and train my associates to use. It has since been applied in NHS outpatient clinics, on digital platforms by a global medical care company and in my own Body Mind Connect online community.

Over the three sections in this book, you will become familiar with the content of this framework for better physical and mental health. Throughout, I will use 'health' as a word to encompass both physical and mental health, reflective of how intertwined they are. Where I need to specify, I will differentiate 'physical' health/illness (e.g. pain, fatigue) from 'psychological' health/illness (e.g. depression, anxiety, stress).

Using this book

I opened Zoom and saw the name of my new client, Reg, in the waiting room. They had just last week made the decision to start sessions with me after noticing a worsening of bowel symptoms since the pandemic restrictions had been lifted, which had only become more troublesome as time went on.

In my usual pre-therapy process, I'd asked him to fill out some forms. As he was particularly keen to get started as soon as possible, I had also given him some pre-session reading: Chapter 1 of the gut-directed cognitive behavioural therapy manual, 'Regul8', which I'd co-authored and that had been used in the biggest research trial to date of therapy for IBS.[3] It was in this trial that we'd received feedback from so many participants, saying, 'If only I had been told this when I was first diagnosed – so much would have been different', over and again. I was quietly hopeful that already the reading would have shifted things slightly for my client.

When I asked him his thoughts about the reading, he told me, 'To be honest I don't care why it's happening, I just want it to stop!'

This made *me* stop and reflect. When you are faced with uncomfortable – sometimes unbearable – symptoms, your brain urgently skips forward to find the metaphorical magic wand. You might be tempted to skip forward in this book to find the action points or the topics that seem most relevant to you. Your brain is quick and tunnel-visioned on the sole aim of alleviation. It can mislead you to assume that more equals better, but that's often not true. Downing a full tub of supplements wouldn't result in quicker healing. Tunnel-vision can lead to overwhelm, frustration, dysregulation and abandoned efforts. The urgency that comes with it can mean your brain skips over important details or dismisses small indications of progress. You may conclude 'another thing that doesn't work for me', when you were on the right lines, you just needed more space and time.

For this reason, I recommend that you read the book in the numerical order of the chapters. Each chapter builds on the last, starting with the mind–body science to help you work with your body effectively. This is where I start with all my clients because it creates empowerment and connection where there has for so long been powerlessness and conflict. When Reg and I spent a session on the physiology of why his bowels were misbehaving, he was jubilant. 'That makes so much sense!'

Having said this, how you read and use this book will depend on where you are broadly in your journey. There are three phases.[4]

- **Crisis:** You are in the midst of uncertainty and disruption. Symptoms/illness may have just started or you are experiencing a sudden worsening, making it hard to find any stability.
- **Coping:** You experience ups and downs, but you have capacity to try things out. You know some things aren't working well and feel you have a lot you would like to change but you are not *completely* overwhelmed and chaotic.
- **Adjustment:** You have found ways to cope and engage with life that work for you. You see room for improvement and growth, but this doesn't feel urgent or frantic. It is explorative, curious and open.

If you are reading this in crisis, give yourself permission to read without needing to do all the exercises. You can come back to them when you feel you are on more solid ground. You might find certain exercises in this book help you get there, but don't put too much pressure on yourself at this stage.

If you are reading this in the coping phase, I suggest you use as many of the exercises as possible. You can pace your reading to match completion of the exercises, or you can simply come back to the exercises when you are ready.

If you are in the adjustment phase, you may like to be more selective over which exercises resonate for where you are or perhaps you can simply take comfort in getting more clarity of the concepts in this book.

The three sections of this book follow the stages I use in my clinical practice.

Section One: Understanding your body
This section introduces you to some fundamental and fascinating mind–body science, covering the key bodily systems that work together to keep you healthy and how they can become dysregulated. This will arm you with important insight into why symptoms start, evolve and keep going from a biopsychosocial perspective and how you can start working with your biology (body) to meet your healing goals.

Section Two: Transforming your experience of symptoms
This section will guide you to map out and personalize your biopsychosocial picture of health, with clarity about what to focus on changing to move towards your healing goals. The practices are designed to help you nurture your mind–body connection and participate in life with joy and meaning.

Section Three: Sustaining changes and becoming who you are
This book aims to provide more than quick hacks that leave you feeling like you're spinning many mini plates to keep everything at bay and OK. This is about making sustainable changes that go beyond singular focus on symptom relief, considering the question of who you are, who you want to be and how to get there. In adversity, there is an opportunity for discovery, and we can cherish this gift without minimizing the cost.

The damage of 'it's all in your head'

My therapy encounter made me feel like my illness was all in my head because the therapist was focussing on my psychological experience without exploring my physical experiences. Beyond inadequately tailored therapy, there are many ways you are told 'it's all in your head' when you get ill or burnt out. Sometimes it's being told 'the tests are normal' and being denied further exploration. Or it can be implied in the unsolicited advice about what you *should* be doing. A big one is generic advice to 'manage your stress'. It can insinuate that symptoms are purely caused by stress, and *you* have control over this stress. Self-help books and social-media content are awash with 'mind over matter' messaging.

I often use a trauma-processing therapy called Eye Movement Desensitization and Reprocessing (EMDR) for physical health issues. I use EMDR not because the health issues are definitively caused by trauma but because the reality of experiencing illness can be traumatic. Your body is bombarded with physical and psychological threats: symptoms, health-related stressors, isolation, life disruption. These threats change how the brain operates, with the threat centres often overactive and the processes for regulating distress and bodily equilibrium inhibited.[5,6,7] EMDR helps to safely consolidate highly distressing past experiences, so that the brain can process the emotion and archive the memory into long-term memory making the present feel safer.[8]

I noticed a definitive theme in the memories being processed by people at their most depleted. They were experiences of receiving the message 'it's all in your head'. In EMDR, you don't process every traumatic or distressing memory. You find the key 'touchstone' memory – that is the memory that encapsulates the core of the emotional distress and/or physical disturbance. So, it was significant that across the many clients I work with, with different conditions, health statuses, life disruptions, and so on, there was such a universal theme that made it hard for the brain to move forward and feel safe.

From these sessions and my wider research, I have distilled what it is about being told 'it's all in your head' that makes it so damaging psychologically and physiologically:

- **Mistrust. You can't trust yourself:** Having your life disrupted, and experiencing immense pain or discomfort and being told that it can't be as bad as you think, or it isn't a 'real' experience, makes you question your sense of reality. This lack of trust of your own mind and body is incredibly destabilizing and creates loops in the brain that further disrupt bodily and emotional regulation (more in Chapter 2).

- **Isolation and disconnection. You're on your own:** In being unheard or disbelieved in your experience, you feel on your own to deal with difficulties. You cannot count on support that you desperately need, making you vulnerable.
- **Over-responsibility. It's all on you:** If others don't accept or understand your experience, it means they cannot help, so you have the sole responsibility for improving things. This creates a host of pressurizing internal assumptions, like you are 100% to blame if you don't recover or if feeling better depends entirely on *you* getting it *right*.

Having 100% responsibility for something, while not being able to trust yourself and not being able to count on necessary support, inhibits you. It also erodes the pillars of safety that your brain and body need to adequately function and regulate. If you resonate and feel a little overwhelmed, don't worry. Breaking down and better knowing the threats now will help to later tailor strategies to increase safety.

According to the Power Threat Meaning Framework (a model developed to better contextualize distress and mental health difficulties in modern-day society), there are six core needs humans have that enable them to feel safe.[9] There is a wealth of research demonstrating that threats to each of these safety domains results in observable changes in your biology.

- **Safe relationships and attachments:** Having positive, stable relationships with caregivers when growing up and as an adult gives you a grounding sense that you will be cared for and helped when needed. This is threatened when you are abandoned by people or experience criticism, dismissal or blame for your own suffering. So significant is the impact of access to relational stability, that a meta-analysis (collation study of a number of other studies and the highest quality research evidence) found that lack of access to stable relationships increased risk of dying by 26% – equivalent to smoking fifteen cigarettes each day.[10]

- **Control/powerlessness:** When you feel powerless to influence your experience, your brain, nervous and immune system functioning changes. A landmark study spanning decades showed that people in jobs with the lowest sense of control had four times the risk of heart disease when compared to colleagues with a high sense of control.[11]
- **Basic physical and material needs:** The brain takes threat to basic safety needs (access to food, water, shelter and protection from harm or health deterioration) seriously. It is evolutionarily ingrained for your body to stay vigilant whilst these threats are present. Long term this can lead to changes in the brain and organs contributing to health deterioration.[12]
- **Sense of fairness and justice about your circumstances:** An awareness of whether you are being treated equally is etched into your biology. Even animals like birds, dogs, donkeys and monkeys have an awareness of fairness and inequality.[13] When you experience injustice or inequality your body can adversely react with dopamine depletion, elevated chronic stress and accelerated aging.[14,15]
- **Being valued:** Feeling that you have significance and are effective in your social roles regulates many internal bodily processes that determine your overall health, including your brain, heart and immune health. Feeling worthless or burdensome can physiologically disrupt focus and motivation, trigger the stress response and increase inflammation.[16]

- **Meaning:** Having hope and a sense of purpose in what you do is often posed societally as a 'nice to have' not a 'must have'. And yet research shows that lacking a sense of meaning or purpose can inhibit the body's ability to feel pleasure, regulate and heal.[17]

My experience with that therapist all those years ago, along with many other experiences of becoming ill around that time (symptoms, healthcare system, time off work), compromised all these core safety needs. My brain was questioning: *How long is it before people get sick of me and give up? What if I never get better? How will I survive if I can't work? Why are things worsening when I am trying so hard? What is the point of me if I'm like this?*

These are common questions that arise when you become ill. Figure 2 illustrates a range of social experiences conveying the message 'it's all in your head'. In turn, these messages violate your core safety needs by eroding your self-trust, pressurizing you beyond your capacity and reducing your sense of support. Violations to these safety needs create biological changes as your body goes into 'threat mode' which can exacerbate physical symptoms.*

You may be surprised to hear that research suggests that the body's *default* biological mode is to anticipate threat at all times.[18] When anticipating threat, specific threat-processing brain areas, like the amygdala and hypothalamus, are activated. These areas constantly make predictions about your safety based on your physical and emotional state and context. Your brain combines this information to communicate with the various bodily networks spanning organs, nerves, hormones and neurotransmitters. Your body is only able to feel safe because it detects markers of safety like being in your home, the access to connection or comfort, the promise of stability, etc. That means when the essence of your

---

* Throughout the book I will use 'symptoms' in relation to physical symptoms or sensations rather than mood or emotional shifts.

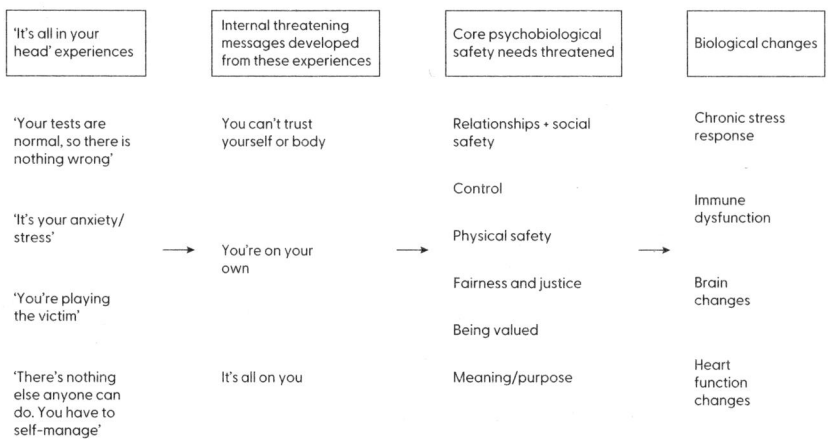

Figure 2: How 'it's all in your head' messages violate core safety needs.

safety is compromised through adversity, ill-health and 'it's all in your head', it can easily become destabilizing. From this place bodily health and mental health can deteriorate.

Reacting to 'it's all in your head'

I've noticed two broad responses to receiving the message 'it's all in your head' illustrated in Figure 3. You may internalize the idea that symptoms and health issues are all your responsibility to figure out and improve. This can result in decision paralysis, because the threat of making the wrong decision is just too huge. Or it can mean that you jump into action and try your hardest to influence everything you have control over. This intense over-responsibility can mean you burn out in your attempts to heal.

On the other end of the spectrum, you may take a defiant stance. 'None of this is in my head, it's all biological processes beyond my control that have nothing to do with psychology!' From here everything becomes pending, until something external changes, further reducing your sense of agency and control. Focussing on psychological aspects of your experience may feel futile or downright insulting.

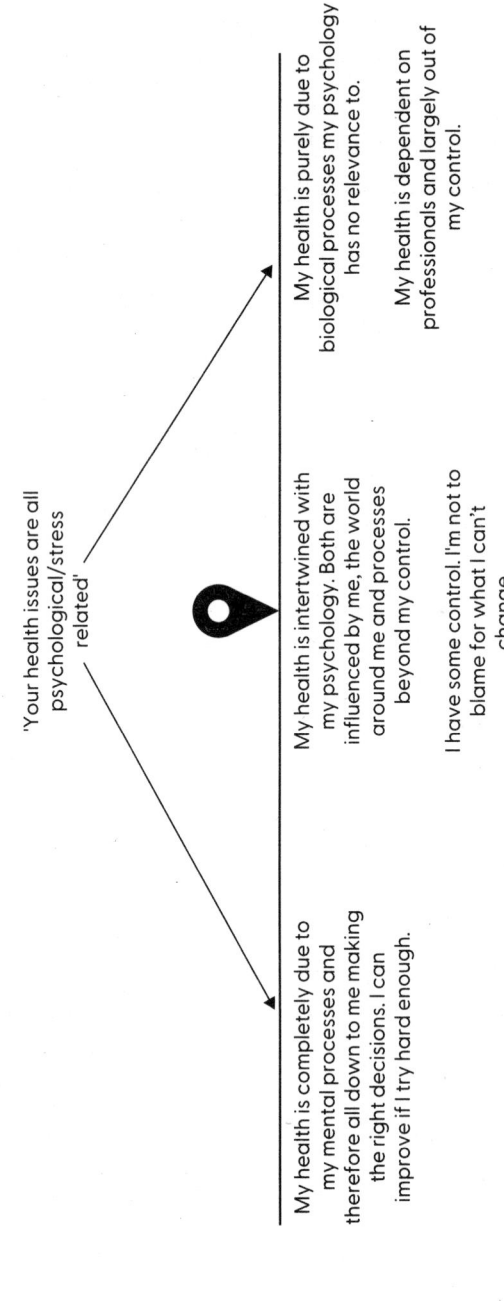

Figure 3: Polarized reactions to 'it's all in your head' and adaptive middle ground.

The dismissive and reductive messaging that health issues are purely caused by your own stress or psychology, means that the role of psychology in health becomes polarized. It is the root cause of *everything* and the answer to everything, *or* it is completely irrelevant. Falling too far on either end of the spectrum leads to disempowerment. It is quite common to ricochet from one end of the spectrum to the other, creating boom/bust patterns which make it harder for your body to regulate (page 154).

The middle ground to safety

When we use psychology to effectively improve health, it's crucial that we move away from messaging that proposes the more in control of your mind you are, the better your health will be. This is a threatening message that can undermine your ability to feel safe.

Biology and psychology are not two opposing ends of the spectrum to be pitched against each other, but are inextricably intertwined in the co-creation of our mental and physical experiences. Mental and physical health is the product of three things that influence each other:

- **Your biology** – your organs, nerves, hormones, etc. that power your everyday experiences
- **Your psychology** – your thoughts, feelings, behaviours, personality and values
- **Your social experiences and environment** – everything from the people around you, to where you live and your day-to-day life.

Figure 4 depicts the well-established framework of health (and life in general), called the Biopsychosocial Model.[19] The premise of this model is that your biology is inseparable from your psychological and social experiences. To have a social experience is to

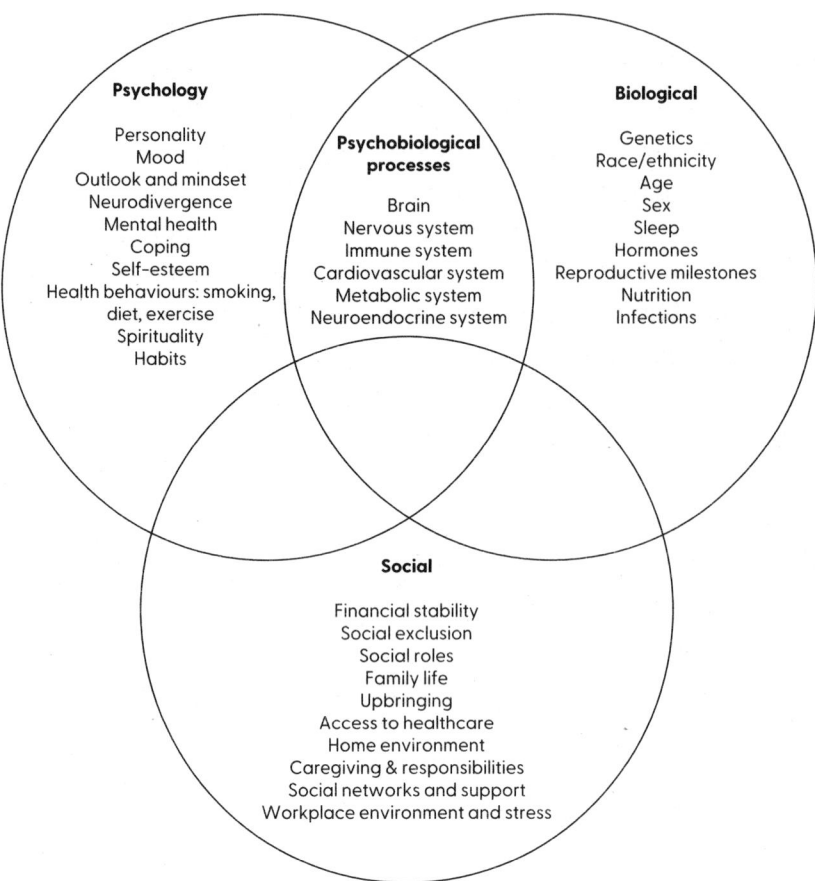

Figure 4: The psychobiological processes that mediate the interaction between biology, psychology and social/environmental experiences with impact on physical health.

also have a psychological and biological (physical) experience, whether or not you are conscious of this.

Let's take the social experience of coming back to work after time off due to illness. This is represented psychologically through thoughts of what you must catch up on, whether anyone resents you for taking time off, emotions (strong or mild) like anticipation, nervousness, or pressure. What you do is informed by these cognitive and emotional processes, further contributing to your psychological experience, such as overworking and feeling more stressed. All of this has biological correlations. Thinking involves electrical and chemical activity in the brain. Feeling anxious or stressed activates the autonomic nervous system. All of these biological processes will be influenced by your baseline physical state, like feeling tired, your immune system working hard to help you heal from illness, disrupted sleep, and so on. Going into work is a seemingly 'simple' experience but it involves multiple mind–body interactions.

In knowing more about the constant conversations between your mind, body and social/environmental experiences, you unlock the potential to restore your sense of safety. The psychotherapeutic framework I created is a biopsychosocial framework, focussing on the intersection between these three spheres to help navigate physical health experiences as well as mood difficulties, trauma, stress and burnout. In the pages of this book, no matter your health or headspace, you will have a flexible framework to meet yourself where you are and move yourself closer to where you want to be.

Setting your own healing goals

Wherever you are in your healing journey, you need to have some kind of orientation to where you want to be. The first step is goal-setting. Don't worry if this feels overwhelming. I'm going to talk you through how to set yourself feasible goals that feel motivating and aligned with your current capacity.

I have seen first-hand how using psychology can create huge transformations, including, but not limited to, complete symptom remission. I've seen people who couldn't conceive because of recurrent infections, go on to have babies after a year or more of being infection-free. Those with extreme pain go on to feel pain no more. I've seen people whose goals were to accept themselves with their disability, go on to shine with a confidence from within. People who made peace with terminal prognoses, living life with meaning and purpose. Often at the start of their journeys, these goals felt anywhere from ambitious to completely unlikely.

When I ask, 'What would you like to be different?', people can struggle to find an answer that is not simply the opposite of what is difficult now: to *not* be in pain, to *have* consistent energy again, to *stop* constantly focussing on sensations. Goals focussed on the absence of something are a shaky foundation on which to make progress because they rely on your brain verifying absence by checking for presence. When your brain checks for the presence of something unwanted it sets off alarm systems in the body. And the more threatened your body feels, the more likely physical symptoms and emotional dysregulation.

At my worst, if someone would have asked me what my goals for healing were, I would have looked at them with disdain as I told them that my goal was to get rid of symptoms and then everything else would be fine. An understandable logic, but the process that will create change is the other way round, which can feel a little back-to-front.

To help you make healing goals, I encourage you to move away from black-and-white symptoms or no symptoms. A beautiful definition of healing comes from *Traditional Healers of Central Australia*,[20] which describes how a Western medical system is complemented by the traditional Ngangkari healers owing to the fact that the Ngangkari healers treat the 'invisible' aspects of illness:

> *Healing is not just about recovering what has been lost or repairing what has been broken. It is about embracing our life force to create a new and vibrant fabric that keeps us grounded and connected, wraps us in warmth and love and gives us the joy of seeing what we have created.*

Healing is more than reclamation of something lost. It is about renewal and discovery. Healing allows you to be at ease, calm and present, no longer flanked by an urgent pressure to outrun or fight some perceived or actual impediment.

> **Pause for a moment. Re-read the quote on healing. Close your eyes. Ask yourself the following questions and write down your answers.**
>
> - What does the word healing mean to you if it is more than specifically getting rid of pain or difficulties?
> - What could embracing your life force look like?
> - What gives you a sense of grounding and connection?
> - What would you like to be doing that you are not doing now?
> - What do you do now that you would stop?
> - How would you be approaching your days? How would you be relating to yourself if you were on your way to heal?

When you have written your answers, read them back through and reflect on what clarity this creates as well as the questions you have. Feel free to come back to this exercise.

Making goals that motivate you

Whatever your goals, we want to move your mind and body out of threat mode, which contributes to the maintaining and/or worsening of symptoms, and towards safety.

This can seem impossible when your body feels hostile and things are uncertain, but during the course of reading this book you'll learn why generating a sense of safety is fundamental to all healing goals and how to get there. I've designed the book so that early on you can have experiences (through doing the exercises) that empower you and feed a sense of hope. Research shows that experiences of empowerment reduce the degree of life disruption from symptoms and physically reduce their severity.[21,22,23] You can then get positive momentum for change as hope and empowerment reduce negative experiences of symptoms, consequently creating more experiences that generate hope and empowerment.

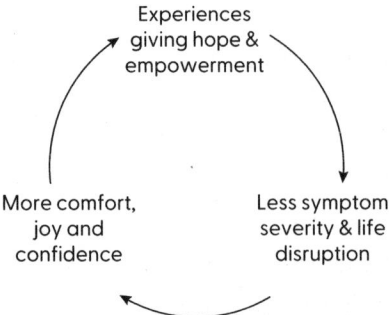

Figure 5: How experiences of empowerment physically reduce symptoms.

To kickstart this, your goals must make you feel hopeful and provide opportunities early on that leave you feeling empowered. This is why I split the goal-setting process into two types of goals:

- **Your big-picture-vision-of-the-future goals (outcome goals).** These goals may not be the 'end' goals, but they are the ones in the distance that may feel far from where you are now.
- **Your stepping-stone goals (process goals).** These goals are focussed on the practice of an action or skill that will contribute towards the end goal. They may be smaller steps that need to be achieved at the start to allow other things to change. For example, being able to interrupt thought spirals day-to-day, is one necessary step that will contribute to reducing anxiety long term.

Where you want to be: big-picture goals

Big-picture goals can generate hope by creating a picture of the future aim/s you have. It is well evidenced that if you have a strong intention with a clear vision, you are more likely to meet that goal (and even surpass it) than if you don't.[24] There is something that can magnify this effect further and that is if you visualize the outcomes. This is not a manifestation myth or woo-woo. It is a well-replicated phenomena that we see in research across disciplines. Using mental imagery can make a huge difference to whether you achieve your goals or not.

One study looked at college students envisaging their day-to-day chores and feeling the sense of accomplishment having done them. Those in the mental imagery group ended up not only doing more but also feeling better about themselves.[25] A similar result was found in tennis players who completed imagery exercises before performing and ended up performing much better than their comparators who had engaged in other pre-performance strategies.[26] The most fascinating of studies I came across was one looking at physical rehabilitation after muscular injuries which had left people in various degrees of immobilization. Participants were instructed to imagine lifting heavy objects at a point where they could not do so physically. Just imagining resulted in increases in muscle strength of up to 136%.[27]

Intentions for getting there: stepping-stone goals

If creating big-picture goals feels too daunting, start with the stepping-stone goals. You can think of these as setting intentions to ground your day-to-day and orient it towards healing. Stepping-stone goals help you to create experiences early in your journey that feel empowering. As well as progressing towards big-picture goals, an important part of their function is to help your brain see proof of progress. Without this, the brain can flail in hopelessness and persuade you there is no point continuing. When this happens, you can find yourself forgetting to do what you set out to do, getting distracted by other things and chasing the novelty of new solutions or promised quick fixes. A big part of my work with people is helping them to see how much they have changed, where their brain has dismissed changes as minimal and meaningless.

The journey is uncertain and can be hard work. Motivation will fluctuate and sometimes entirely leave you, and so you can't rely on that alone. You need to teach yourself to recognize and value the 'small' markers of progress along the way. Studies show that monitoring and acknowledging the small successes, increases your chances of meeting your goals and enhances your ability to stick with habits.[28]

The rise in interest about 'manifestation' has seen misinformation spread like wildfire about how all you need to do is believe and visualize that belief. This is categorically untrue (I'm sorry!). When people who manifest were compared to people who don't believe in manifestation, they were no more likely to reach their goals.[29] In one study, researchers found that the opposite was true. Those who relied on manifestation through visualization were less likely than their non-manifesting counterparts to reach their goals.[30] The authors also measured the degree of effort expended towards the goals. Those who believed strongly in the power of thought and visualization tended to expend less effort.

This reminds me of the joke about the person who dies, meets God at the pearly gates and says, 'I prayed all my life, went to church and here I am in Heaven, but why, Lord, did you not grant me my hopes of winning the lottery?' To which God replies, 'Well, I tried, but you never bought a lottery ticket!'

Setting your goals

Goal-setting can be done in stages. I recommend at this stage you start creating clarity on your big-picture outcome goals. Once you have more understanding on what the processes are that will help get you there, you can start creating tailored stepping-stone process goals. There will be an invitation to do so throughout the book. I've included some examples of outcome and process goals that this book can help you to implement (Table 1).

Table 1: Goal-setting guidance		
Outcome goal type	**Outcome goal example**	**Process goal examples**
Reducing or eliminating symptoms	To have 0% pain most of the days of the week	• To observe my thoughts when in pain rather than get stuck on the worst-case scenario • To focus on comfort not fixing things when in severe pain
	To feel energized and alert during the daytime most days of the week	• To pace my activities so that I don't over-exert myself too often • To assert myself when I need to say 'no'
Increasing capabilities or engagement in life	To be able to see friends for dinner	• To increase food variety when at home • To disclose food concerns to trusted friends
	To be able to work seven-hour days	• To take regular breaks to minimize over-exertion and allow for four-hour days • To recognize signs of burnout early to allow for replenishment
Reducing emotional discomfort	To feel less anxious day-to-day	• To interrupt worry spirals earlier and contemplate neutral and positive outcomes • To tune into my body and use practices to calm it

	To feel more pleasure and less sadness each day	• To meet self-critical thoughts with compassion • To prioritize connecting with others each week
Increasing or enhancing confidence or connection with self	To feel more confident in my ability to handle difficult things	• To log hard things I have overcome • To explore skills and abilities of mine that I naturally overlook
	To stop seeing myself as weak or a failure	• To process and update past experiences contributing to this narrative • To log my successes and things I deserve credit for

Throughout the book you will become familiar with all the concepts touched upon with these process goals (and more) and how they nurture the mind–body connection in chronic illness, burnout and recovering from trauma. You can have multiple process goals for each outcome goal because healing is never down to just one thing. This gives you flexibility.

Goal-setting and perfectionism

Perfectionism isn't the pursuit of perfect. It is the pursuit of unrelenting standards or rules that aim to make you feel good enough, safe or in control. Throughout this book, we are going to challenge and play with automatic perfectionist tendencies. When goal-setting, perfectionism can make you believe that you need to have the most rigorous and well-informed goals that account for all the various strands of the issue/s you face. However, the reality is that in therapy we tend to make a rough start with a broad idea of big-picture outcome/s and some ideas of how to get there. We refine as we go. There will be lots of opportunity for doing this throughout the book.

> **For now, ask yourself:**
>
> - What is my biggest difficulty (difficulties)? Get as specific as you can with what it/they are and how they affect you.
> - Specifying outcome goals: What would it look like in 3, 6 or 12 months' time for this difficulty to be improved (in whatever way you like or think could be feasible)? Again, get as specific as you can. Try and focus on what would be happening or possible, rather than what is no longer there (although this can be hard, so you can start with the absence of something and then ask, if that wasn't there – what would I be doing or feeling instead of now?).
> - Identifying process goals: What sorts of things would you like to be able to do or stop doing that you think could help get you closer to your outcome goals? You can start generally, without knowing exactly how you can achieve these things. For example, I will be calmer when I have symptoms. You can also list several options.
>
> For each outcome goal, rate out of 10 how close you are to that goal now, with zero not at all and 10 completely. We'll come back to this as we go.

What you can hope for

Everything in this book is written to help you and your body move from a default of threat, doom and powerlessness to safety, hope and empowerment. Whether you are struggling with health or mood difficulties that have a clear or unknown origin, in the pages of this book you will learn how to work with your psychology and biology to meet your healing goals.

As you become familiar with the ways that the internalized trope, 'it's all in your head', creates pressure, urgency and self-blame, undermining your ability to heal, you will also come to know the choices, compassion and transformation offered when you realize it's all in your body. What dwells in the mind, dwells in the body. From here, you can feel open to try out new approaches without the fear of getting it wrong or being optionless if they don't work. You can gain comfort in finding ways to bring richness and meaning to your life *now*, rather than putting life on hold to heal.

By the end of the book, you will find yourself clearer on and closer to your healing goals and yourself. The latter is necessary for the former.

People come to me as a last-ditch attempt to physically and emotionally heal. They've seen all the specialist doctors, tried the supplements, followed restrictive diets and still they suffer. There's just one missing piece, or at least that's what it feels like. And mostly, people aren't all that convinced that seeing a health psychologist is that missing piece, but then what other options have they got?

'Just to let you know, doc, I am sceptical.'

I hear this a lot and it makes me smile. I'm not smiling with self-importance or arrogance that I have the answer. It's one of enduring warmth and recognition of a fellow human experiencing the curse (and gift) of human brain processes. Of course you're sceptical.

I smile because you are sceptical and still you come. You try and you suspend your scepticism and lean into your curiosity and hope. There is strength in that. There is transformation in that.

I smile because, just now, we have started a journey together. We have decided to team up and explore the pieces of what has come before, to work out how we shape what comes next for the better. This is a brave move and for many it can feel extremely vulnerable. Admitting the need for help and opening up so much in order to get it. I'm smiling at the connection and unity that there is in that.

A moment from when I was at my most ill comes back to me from time to time. It's like I am watching myself, a blurred still frame on me, while all around me everything is colourful and dynamic. At the time, I was sitting on the couch at a relative's home and everyone seemed light and carefree. They spoke to each other melodically, while I remained still and monosyllabic. Outside I was frozen, but inside everything was racing with panic and resentment. *How could they go on like this when I was so broken? Why was I so broken?*

At one point it got too much. The swell of internal dialogue made me feel intensely self-conscious and out of place. I broke down in tears and ran out of the house. I had nowhere to go. I had no car, and I couldn't walk very far because I was depleted and sore. I ended up sitting on a neighbour's wall and crying. Moments later, my dad came out, his expression incredulous and impatient. He pulled me off the wall as my sobs turned to wails. He didn't understand why I'd run out. And I was appalled that he didn't understand.

My husband wrote a song about that version of me and what might have been had I remained buried by all the pain and hopelessness. It's called Hollow.

She told me she was hollow, that's far from what I see.

This one line is the antithesis of that moment. It is being seen in your deepest moments of internal anguish, when on the outside you are a blurry still frame.

The song went on to connect with millions of people worldwide and I believe that's because it touches on our core need to be seen and heard when we are at our most vulnerable.

I hope this chapter has helped to clarify that illness, burnout and mood issues are not all in your head. That the interaction between mind and body can be understood from a biopsychosocial model of health. And that even goal-setting involves working with your mind and body, with a clearer idea of how to start this process to meet your healing goals.

Wherever you are in your journey, let me reassure you that I have not met one person I've worked with who had no scope for hope. Your brain can try and protect you from getting your hopes up, and that can close down hope and experimentation. That's where I was. But just as I am now so far from that 'hollow girl', you too can be far from your equivalent. Just as I smile with my patients at the start of their journeys, I am smiling with you for the start of yours and the depths of empowerment you have yet to uncover.

SECTION ONE

Understanding your body

'Just knowing why my body is reacting like this, has changed everything. I don't freak out now. I can even comfort it and see symptoms fade'
– Quote from a patient with multiple diagnoses

When you picture healing, what do you see? Perhaps you imagine yourself enjoying a bright blue sky, feeling the sun on your skin, as you walk uninterrupted by symptoms. Or clicking the 'confirm' button to book flights for a holiday, feeling nothing but excitement at the prospect, confident that a flare-up won't stop you. Or perhaps it's finding calm stillness in a frantic mind.

Whatever you imagine, the likelihood is that you are picturing yourself *taking action.*

As a health psychologist and psychotherapist, I work with people whose lives are disrupted by symptoms. When clients start working with me, they are ready to make change and are awaiting direction. That direction needs to be informed by an understanding of what is making *now* so difficult and how this is influenced by the mind–body connection. That is where we'll start in this book.

Section One will build a solid foundation of knowledge about how your mind and body communicate and, specifically, how this communication affects you physically, mentally and emotionally.

This section of the book is going to help you:

- Better understand yourself and your experience of symptoms
- Create healing goals
- Recognize patterns that keep you stuck in symptom spirals
- Generate ideas for interrupting those patterns.

You will no doubt feel the pressure to *make change*, but be patient with yourself. Just by reading, you are changing your brain. And changes in the brain pave the way for changes in the body.

CHAPTER 1

Befriending your biology

In the waiting rooms of sexual health clinics, GP surgeries and specialist urogynaecology wards, I would sit subdued, not knowing if I would finally receive an answer about why I was feeling so awful. At the beginning of my illness, there was more certainty, as old male doctors threw definitive diagnoses and treatment regimens at me. As things went on and nothing worked, I seemed to morph in their eyes from a weak and over-anxious young girl getting het up over a run-of-the-mill infection, to a complex problem patient. The shrugging of shoulders, the raising of eyebrows, the avoidance of eye contact and the fixed concentration on computer screens, all told me that what was happening to me had no easy fix. There was *one* definitive though: stress. Specifically, that I should avoid it because it would only make things worse. This was a cruel irony, because feeling so physically awful was inherently stressful. How, exactly, should I go about avoiding it?

Something else was changing too. My belief that I could be helped was rapidly diminishing. The less the medical system was able to help me, the more disconnected I felt from those around me. No one understood my experience. I also had a growing sense that people were thinking that I was the one responsible for all of this. That I was causing it or making it up. My skin prickled at the slightest impatience or dismissal from others, as though I was creating a forcefield to protect me from the unspoken accusations. All of this made me question my sanity and hate my body – it always seemed to react in the 'wrong' way. I'd dread the suggestion of new medications because I was sure to have a bad reaction.

Although stress does interact with your biology, often the messaging around it can elicit the three central threats of 'it's all in your head': that you are on your own, that it's yours to fix, and that you cannot trust your body. This chapter will give you an understanding of your biology and the body's regulatory systems, so that you can shed the burden of over-responsibility for illness and re-establish some confidence in your body's ability to help you out. You will gain new insight into how your body reacts to stress and threat, and how you can start to work with some of these biological processes to coax your mind and body back to a sense of safety. Importantly, by the end of this chapter, you will recognize that feeling unfixable is a narrative from a threatened brain and not a reality. As you become more familiar with the mind–body dynamics detailed in this chapter, you will be more empowered to befriend your biology. The information in this chapter creates a foundation for enacting that befriending, which Section Two will go on to describe.

Your stress, your fault?

We've all been there – reading articles or consuming webinars about all the ways *you* can better manage *your* stress, only adding to your mental to-do list and creating more stress. Stress management messaging can make stress feel like a personal failing. This issue is intensified if you find yourself impacted by illness. Stress is a big factor in health. It can vastly change wound healing, recovery from illness, gut microbiomes and more.[1] Many of my patients tell me that they are stressed about being stressed. This means when they experience stress, they immediately get an additional layer of stress, worrying that it will make their symptoms worse. This can result in all kinds of strategies to try to avoid stress, which – spoiler alert – tend to make things worse and *more* stressful. Research shows that when you view stress as less of a threat, your body is physiologically better able to regulate the stress response, with benefits for your physical health, symptoms and mental wellbeing.[2,3,4]

So, how can you feel less threatened by stress?

It helps to break down what 'stress' means because the word has multiple meanings:

- **Stress as a stressor.** 'I have so much stress right now' describes someone experiencing multiple stressors (things that are stressing you). These can be external things like deadlines, arguments and noisy neighbours, or internal things like worries about the future or the pressure to achieve. Many stressors are outside of our control.
- **Stress as an automatic response.** 'I am so stressed out' refers to the experience of stress psychologically and/or physiologically. This is the stress response to stressors you are experiencing. You may identify with stress purely as the psychological experience which can feel like anxiety or agitation – although not always – but the physical stress response can occur even without feeling psychologically stressed. More on this in a moment.
- **Stress as an action.** 'I am *stressing* out' describes a reaction to stress. Stress reactions might be observable like pacing about or involve internal processes like repetitive thinking about problems.

The degree of control we have over each type of stress varies, as does the degree of helpfulness in *trying* to reduce the different types of stress. Trying to eradicate stressors is generally implausible, although there may be room to mitigate some. Trying not to feel stressed when you feel stressed can have variable results, often making stress feel even more overwhelming.

It is the 'stress actions' (reactions to stress) that can influence the degree of threat from stress. Think of moments like mentally revisiting all the things that you might have done wrong in a test or meeting new friends. Or when you meticulously check everything is accounted for before committing to any plans. In the coming chapters we'll look at how changing your reactions to stress can reduce the degree of threat from stress. One thing you need to know is that having imperfect automatic reactions to difficult things is human and generally unavoidable. Stress can make you more reactive, and/or less able to react. It can mean that you lash out or act impulsively, making decisions that in hindsight didn't serve you. That is OK. What matters is how you meet yourself after these moments, in the hours, days and months that follow. Meeting yourself with awareness, curiosity and compassion counts for a lot when it comes to working with your biology. This can sound like a simple acknowledgement of, 'I'm finding this really overwhelming, and I need a minute.' Or it can look like a calm regrouping, as you decide the next action that will serve you (and your relationships) better.

Reduce stress micromanagement

When you repeatedly hear how harmful stress is, you may feel the burden of trying to undo any harm stress might have caused. This can lead to attempts to 'micromanage' stress by avoiding it or by trying to immediately counteract it. The internet is now awash with ways to 'hack your vagus nerve' and 'regulate your nervous system'. This can encourage the expectation that you should immediately take a break from anything that increases stress and/or seek to counterbalance all stress you encounter. These expectations can build fearful beliefs about stress, activity and emotions. These fears and these responses to stress can disrupt rather than enhance bodily balance.

Trying to relax during intense stress can be frustrating and demoralizing, because your biological systems are working in the other direction. That's why it is important for you to know how your biological systems work during stress. This can reduce the threat of stress and help you work with your body more effectively to reduce stress. Many of my clients with panic disorder have found that just knowing what is happening in their body when they experience extreme palpitations, can be enough to stop the panic attack in its tracks, so that they no longer fear an imminent heart attack.

The stress response has two dedicated biological pathways. One is a more immediate 'quick-fire' response to stress that activates in moments like realizing you are about to miss your train or that a child is running into a road. The other is a more 'sustained stress response' that continues over a longer duration, like when you have an upcoming deadline that you have to keep working towards, or if you are a carer for a relative who has ongoing needs. The two pathways are often conflated in messaging about stress being bad for your health, making you fear your quick-fire stress response. In those moments where you get breathless in an argument or get a shaky anticipation before seeing friends, your brain may associate this as harmful for your body. You may pull back from things that are really important for you to do for your mood and bodily balance – as we'll see later.

Quick-fire stress response

The quick-fire stress response is better known as fight or flight (or freeze). It occurs because of a sequence of communications in a pathway called the sympathetic-adreno-medullary (SAM) system. Let's say you have a heart flutter, your brain may detect this as a threat without you having a conscious thought. A region of your brain called the hypothalamus has activated your autonomic nervous system (ANS). This is the part of your nervous system that is dedicated to many automatic bodily responses including your bowel and bladder function. This is why you can find yourself needing the toilet more urgently when you are nervous. Specifically, the sub-branch of the ANS, called the sympathetic nervous system (SNS), activates.

Activation of the SNS results in the release of activating hormones like adrenaline and noradrenaline into the bloodstream. This biological process allows you to meet demands. If you are sitting on the couch ensconced in a movie and someone comes in and asks for your help in the kitchen, it is the SNS that will activate to help you switch gears, get up and do what needs to be done. In heightened stress, the level of activation is greater. The greater the stress, the greater the release of hormones. When these hormones are in the bloodstream, they bind to receptors on your muscles and organs, changing how they are functioning so that they can be primed for action. This is why you might feel the physical need to move when anxious. In Chapter 3, you'll get more familiar with how the SNS influences specific symptoms.

Sustained stress response

The sustained stress response is communicated across another biological pathway, called the hypothalamic-pituitary-adrenal (HPA) axis. The SAM system and the HPA axis are well-trodden routes in the body to communicate messages relating to stress, demands and threats. The HPA axis 'route' can activate at the same time as the SAM system, but it takes slightly longer to engage. Bodily changes that occur as a result of the HPA activation are therefore slower to elicit and more gradually conducted. Rather than a rapid bowel spasm that might happen when your quick-fire stress response kicks in, the changes happening in your body due to the sustained stress response are less experientially discernible at a given moment.

It is the changes that happen more gradually under the surface due to HPA activation/dysregulation that are responsible for the negative impacts of stress on health. But before you despair, there is comfort in this. I will illustrate by using two household malfunctions. Quick-fire stress (SAM system) is like a drain in the garden getting blocked and causing a stench and some flooding. It causes instant and obvious disruption. It is unpleasant, but ultimately unblocking is simple, sometimes happening spontaneously should rain wash away the blockage. Sustained stress (HPA axis) is like a very slow gas leak. There may be no signs, no smell and no real symptoms until it gets to a level over a long period of time where the room is saturated with gas.

To protect yourself from a gas leak, you don't have to constantly check the boiler and take new readings of air purity, but you do need regular boiler maintenance and a clear alarm system that alerts you if gas increases to a noxious level. This is the same with cumulative stress, yet most of us don't have clarity on our alarm systems, which are often only alerted when the body is severely impacted.

Now for all those anxious brains reading this, the secretions of the sustained stress response are not deadly like carbon monoxide! When the sustained stress response is active, it results in a release of the stress hormone cortisol, which has been a tad unfairly demonized. Cortisol allows your body to sustain the stress response by maintaining blood sugar levels, regulating energy and sensitizing your body to adrenaline and noradrenaline. This helps you stay alert and active to deal with your stressors, such as carrying on working to meet your deadline or maintaining focus on a long drive. The sensitization to adrenaline and noradrenaline is also one of the reasons why you may end up feeling more reactive to small stressors when you are dealing with ongoing stress or why you can feel wired and hyper-alert when everything else in you is telling you that you need to switch off.

Your body's natural stress counterbalance

Your body has an inbuilt counterbalance to the quick-fire stress response: the parasympathetic nervous system (PNS). The PNS activates to clear excess adrenaline and restore normal bodily function. The vagus nerve is the main nerve of the PNS. It carries signals between the brain and major organs, including your heart, lungs, digestive system, bladder and more. When the PNS is activated, the vagus nerve slows your heart rate, restores digestion, reduces inflammation, and releases calming neurotransmitters like acetylcholine, helping your body to recover and rebalance. Generally, you don't have to do anything for this process to naturally take place. In the moments where you are feeling highly stressed, perhaps awaiting a medical appointment, or the outcome from a test, you have options to stimulate this natural counterbalance to help calm the body (more in Chapter 4).

The best thing you can do to buffer against the negative long-term effects of the sustained stress response is to play the slow long game. Much like investments, focussing on short-term gains tends to make for a much less stable trajectory of returns, whereas consistently putting away what you can afford tends to favour longer-term stability. With stress, this means taking the pressure off yourself to escape or avoid stress when it arises, and instead to cultivate sustainable habits and support systems that can hold you when your stress and health fluctuates (like the stock market). More on this in Chapter 5.

The bodily balancing act

With the rise of content out there about 'dysregulated nervous systems' it is important to clarify the concept here. It refers to an imbalance of the ANS functioning so that the body's ability to naturally counterbalance stress, as described above, is inhibited. The concept comes from Polyvagal Theory and there is some good science demonstrating that the ANS can become dysregulated due to chronic stress and trauma.[5]

This is where clarification in terminology is important. The term 'dysregulated nervous system' does not specify *which* nervous system is dysregulated. The ANS is only one branch of a much larger nervous system, which is divided into two: the central nervous system and the peripheral nervous system. The brain is the key component of the central nervous system, along with the spinal cord, integrating information from your body, your environment, and coordinating your responses (emotional, physical and cognitive). The brain receives information from the rest of the body through the network of nerves that make up your peripheral nervous system.

The ANS is a sub-branch of the peripheral nervous system. If you hurt your hand, the nerves in your hand send messages up to your brain, which will process the signals to produce what your experience is (e.g. pain and panic or lack of sensation and nonchalance). Dysregulation in how your brain processes this, as well as dysregulation in the communication between your brain, spinal cord and nerves, can result in more pain, more difficult-to-explain symptoms like fatigue and a tendency to have multiple physical symptoms.[6,7]

Your brain also receives information from your body and distributes instructions to it, via four key internal regulatory systems that are responsible for navigating your body back to a state of balance and stability, called homeostasis (Figure 6).[8] These regulatory systems coordinate everything from basic functions to keep you alive (breathing, sleeping, digesting) to sophisticated processes like healing from injury or illness, or emotionally and physically regulating in or after extreme stress.

These regulatory systems are:

- **The neuroendocrine system.** The communication network between your brain and hormones that regulates multiple bodily functions including energy use

and the stress response. The ANS works closely with this system.
- **The immune system.** Your body's defence against infections and injuries. It fights off harmful bacteria, infections and damaged cells, repairs tissue and manages inflammation to keep you healthy.
- **The cardiovascular system.** Your heart, blood vessels and blood that deliver oxygen and nutrients to your body and get rid of waste, adjusting heart rate and blood pressure in response to increased bodily demands (e.g. physical activity or stress).
- **The metabolic system.** Your body's energy management system including processes like digestion, blood sugar control and fat storage. It is responsible for converting food into energy and stores or releases it as needed, ensuring your cells get enough energy to perform their functions.

The regulatory systems negotiate bodily balance by working out what adjustments need to be made in the face of changing conditions (like your environment, your mood, stressors, injury, etc.). The smallest condition shift can result in change in regulatory processes. For example, when the temperature drops, a whole sequence of communications from the brain (specifically the hypothalamus) to the metabolic system via the ANS and neuroendocrine system, allows your body to prioritize heat production and enhance energy efficiency to keep you at a healthy temperature for your organs to function.

While your regulatory systems maintain balance, your health remains intact, and you have access to the energetic resources you need. Each system is inherently resilient, having a natural ability to rebalance. The dynamic between the systems allows further leeway, so that if one system is impeded, the other(s) can compensate so that you may not even know the difference.

Take the example of menstruation. Each regulatory system

contributes towards keeping the body functioning healthily around this change in physiology. The cardiovascular system can compensate for excess blood loss by constricting blood vessels to maintain blood pressure. The neuroendocrine system regulates hormones that naturally fluctuate during menstruation, ensuring that there is not a prolonged cortisol response. The metabolic system regulates nutrient levels by increasing cravings and making more glucose available where necessary. The immune system manages the inflammatory response to protect against infection while tissues in the uterus break down. This is a beautiful example of how your body is constantly working to keep all these systems stable – and 99% of the time you don't even notice, precisely because it is brilliantly performing so many jobs. The significance of these regulatory systems in nurturing the mind–body connection will become clearer throughout the coming chapters. You have the potential to directly affect each bodily system pictured in Figure 6. This gives you the potential power to create a positive ripple effect across the bodily systems through your actions and mental processing.

A threatened brain is a threatened body

Your brain has the ginormous task of integrating messages from the various nervous systems and regulatory systems (Figure 6). You may recall that the body's default biological setting is to anticipate and quickly react to threat (threat mode).[9] This is underpinned by the key threat-processing areas of the brain (amygdala and hypothalamus). Balance across bodily systems is maintained when your brain detects less threat and perceives more safety. For this to happen, it needs to be able to attend to cues of safety, like affection, being cared for, feeling connected, having autonomy, choice or influence. These cues can become scarcer when you get ill. Your brain's ability to detect them is also inhibited by the biological stress responses. For you, this may feel like an

Top Down

We can work with psychological experiences processed predominantly in the brain to generate more psychological safety. This will have a positive downstream effect on processes in the regulatory systems and nervous system, to allow more access to physiological equilibrium.

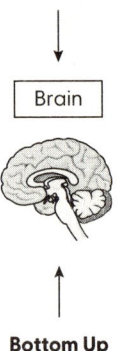

Bottom Up

We can work with physical experiences somatically and through changes to behaviour to more directly alter dysregulation in the regulatory systems and nervous systems. This helps create safety signals in the body with an 'upstream' soothing effect to the brain and broader psychological experience.

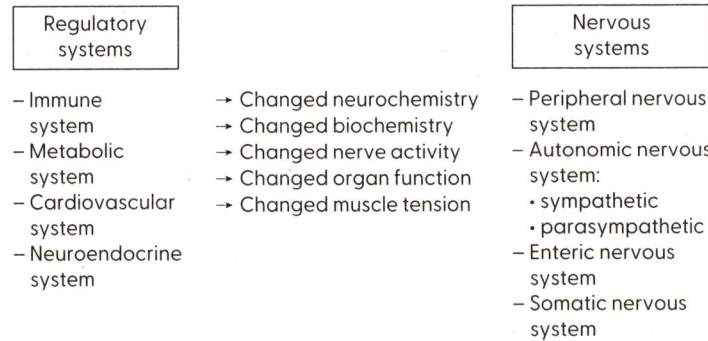

Figure 6: The interconnectivity between the brain and bodily systems and scope for influencing them for better health.

utter lack of control as your brain keeps dragging your attention to things that make you feel bad or sad, and when you try to look at things from another perspective it doesn't feel believable. Thinking can't always change how you feel when you're in threat mode. Here's why.

An area of your brain called the prefrontal cortex (PFC) acts as a central control centre for your mind, in charge of your attention, ability to hold information, problem-solve and more. It plays a chief role in regulating your emotions. It does this by communicating with the emotion- and threat-processing centres to reduce activation, which you experience as a calming down. However, when things are particularly threatening or distressing, activation in these emotion-processing areas is heightened and these brain areas communicate with other centres in the brain and body (including the SAM system and HPA axis), reducing the PFC's ability to calm things. In these moments, it is often more effective to work with the body to calm down the brain activity, by cultivating experiences that provide a sense of safety (more in Chapter 5). You can get stuck in a loop of trying to think to feel better, only to find the thoughts generate more difficult feelings. Threat mode has changed how your brain is working, meaning the usual strategies (e.g. trying to think things through) are producing different results (e.g. feeling worse).

Trauma and the brain

When you experience extreme distress or trauma, this 'amygdala hijack' can have longer-term changes because it affects how your brain remembers things. An inhibited PFC and highly activated amygdala and hippocampus means that the intense emotionality of your experience is imprinted to memory so that it can easily be recalled. In extreme trauma, such as post-traumatic stress disorder (PTSD), this can result in vivid intrusive memories of traumatic experiences. When you become ill, distressing experiences (whether or not you regard them as traumatic) can similarly be imprinted.

Vivid feelings and urges to escape can be triggered (e.g. by symptoms) without specific memories attached. The hippocampus usually consolidates memories, combining new experiences with prior ones and existing knowledge. In extreme distress or trauma, it is prevented from doing so, creating easily elicited but fragmented memories. In this sense, your brain gets 'stuck' at the point of past distress. This is why you may dread going to the doctor's even though you know you are only going for cough medication, but previously you were fighting for a diagnosis. The brain elicits that same dread of powerlessness, even though the context is quite different. All of this can generate a sense of mistrust in yourself, your reactions, your sense of reality and your ability to soothe yourself when feeling intense emotions.

Hopefully knowing a little about how your brain may process things will help you feel less at fault for things you may have been struggling with. Perhaps it will also give you some ideas about what scope there is for helping to update the brain and cultivate a sense of much-needed safety. When you know what is happening in the brain, you are much better equipped to work with it to make lasting change. Don't worry, Section Two will show you how to do this explicitly.

Establishing trust after dysregulation

As your body is constantly multitasking across these interconnected networks in the background to keep you hydrated, nourished and responsive to threats (e.g. infections, stressors), it is understandable that maintaining balance will not always be possible. You might experience this imbalance in the form of out-of-the-blue symptoms like persistent fatigue or recurrent colds or increased anxiety. To you, the conscious human at the helm of a highly automated biological ship, it feels completely unexpected and it creates more threat. You may scrutinize what is happening. Perhaps focussing on what your body feels like or second-guessing the reason for symptoms cropping up. You might intuitively try to help, adding things into the mix, like more medications or supplements. Or taking things out of the mix by reducing activity or avoiding certain foods.

I think of this process like a manager that suddenly steps in after a major error. Until the point of error, the team has been functioning well. Outputs have been on target and the team has gone largely unnoticed for all they've been doing. And yet after the error, the manager assumes the whole team is useless and has been doing *everything* wrong. The manager starts overhauling all sorts of protocols without fully understanding how that will affect other elements of the work on the floor and then when there are negative repercussions from that, the manager blames the team. During this process, trust between team and manager is eroded. Much like it is for you and your body. This is why it is important that you know a little about the processes that disrupt your bodily balance and how they come about.

Disruption to your regulatory systems' ability to come back to balance (homeostasis) regularly, is called allostatic load.[10] Your body can be prevented from reaching homeostasis by too much or too little demand on these regulatory systems. Excess *ongoing* stress without adequate buffers can create too much demand. The bodily mistrust and micromanagement can add substantially to this demand. Other examples of too much additional demand are things like lifestyle factors (e.g. drinking or smoking), medically unmanaged illness or injury or excess repeated physical exertion (e.g. running on an injury). When there is too much demand, your systems are swamped with more work than they can handle. Too little demand means that your systems aren't 'worked out' enough to maintain their adaptability and resiliency for challenges. A lack of physical activity or mental stimulation are examples of too little demand. So too (perhaps surprisingly) is a lack of stress. You need healthy doses of stress to keep your systems trained and flexible.

One of the reasons it can be so hard to regain trust between you and your body after dysregulation is because there isn't a clear dichotomy of good versus bad things for rebalancing. It is about the act of balancing. Sleep is an example of this. When you get a virus, you may naturally require more sleep. Getting that extra sleep is necessary for your regulatory systems to rebalance. However, too much sleep will inhibit recovery, because excessive sleep can lower overall metabolic activity, slowing the circulation of immune cells and inhibiting lymphatic drainage, increasing inflammation. So how do you work out when is too much sleep if you continue to feel tired and not completely well? The uncertainty of the balancing act can lead to more stress, more allostatic load and longer recovery time.

Part of re-establishing trust with your body is learning to step away from the generalized sense that it is doing everything wrong. This means recognizing where your body has been coping with additional demands or has been impeded, sometimes even by your well-intentioned efforts to help. To illustrate this, I'll share a bit of Heather's story.

Heather's story

Heather could not understand why her quality of life was changing every day. There was no clear reason why she would wake up one morning feeling unwell and different from her usual self, and then the next day feel OK. It had been two years since her symptoms had started 'out of the blue' and they had never receded. In fact, they had worsened to the point that she could no longer work.

Her symptoms started with severe body aches and tingles, that felt viral, but had morphed into a vast array of physical symptoms. Doctors perceived these symptoms as unusual and often shrugged them off as 'just stress'. Yes, she did feel stressed, she conceded, but this was because of the bodily symptoms she was experiencing. They were sometimes so debilitating all she could do was lie down, head spinning, heart racing.

When she found me, she had been searching for the puzzle piece that would make sense of her symptoms. She was mildly hopeful but generally resigned. She was a medical mystery that had exhausted every corner of the biomedical system. The more apparently mysterious her symptoms were, the more she had the sense that she was destined to be stuck for ever. As we talked, I took in her drawn face and the sadness in her eyes, slightly glazed as she tried to communicate just how hard she had tried. She explained her story, bracing herself to be told once again that this was all 'in her head'. I promised her that we would unpack her experience so that it was no longer unknowable and importantly no longer felt completely unfixable. Knowing what her body had been contending with would give her important insights into what it needed to feel safe again and to healthily rebalance. In the next sections, I'll help you break down your own experiences, with reference back to Heather.

Three phases of becoming unwell

There are three phases that influence the development of health* issues (Figure 7):

- Pre-birth and early years
- The run-up period (to illness onset or symptom worsening)
- Triggering phase

---

* Applies to mental health issues and burnout too

Some phases may have more significance than others depending on your illness/symptoms. At each phase, violations to the six core safety needs (safe relationships/attachment, control, basic physical needs, sense of fairness or justice, being valued, and having meaning) can contribute to allostatic load.

There are some experiences that you have no control over – some even before you were born. The good news is that you don't need a time-machine to undo the things that have contributed to allostatic load. Just being able to acknowledge their impact can help increase bodily safety and open choices in the present. Neuroscience research shows that acknowledgement and awareness of past 'threats' can physiologically change processes in the brain.[11,12] Where the brain may have learnt helplessness, retracing the past from a different lens with new knowledge can create hope and reduce automatic threat activation. In this section, you'll be guided to acknowledge what these threats or stressors might have been for you. In Section Two of this book, you'll be supported to help re-establish safety.

Pre-birth and early years

Your regulatory systems are affected by the allostatic demands of your parents and grandparents because of the genes you inherit and something called epigenetics. Your genes are the manuals that are embedded in the cells that make up your body and tell them how to work, affecting your bodily function and psychology. Genes aren't static. They are subject to updates based on life experiences: the contact you have with pathogens, injuries or ailments, stress or trauma, the environment you live in. All of this has the potential to interact with your genetic coding. This is epigenetics.

Once born, you go through critical periods of brain development in childhood and adolescence, where your brain is quicker to absorb information. These rapid brain changes impact your allostatic functioning. If you experience lots of stress or threat in childhood or adolescence, your regulatory systems will experience more demands changing how your body is functioning.[13] Childhood bullying, exclusion, illness, parental separation, heated arguments, or cold-shouldering (of partner, child or siblings) and excessive alcohol consumption of caregivers all constitute threats that influence regulatory system functioning.

Heather initially told me how 'normal' her childhood was. Upon exploring, she shared that she had been hospitalized in primary school after contracting glandular fever and then meningitis. She remembered being scared and confused. She was held back at school because of the health complications, concluding that she was more fragile than other children who she would see playing carefree whilst she felt isolated by the burden of knowing what *could* go wrong. Heather's cells were at their most malleable when all these things were happening. Although for many years these experiences had been forgotten, they were immediately remembered by the body when it sensed a similar thing was happening again. Part of the body remembering was the activation of threat responses.

Recognizing this played an important role in helping her body to feel safe again as she grappled with new symptoms. The 'unfixable' lens had been activated, and we had to create opportunities to switch off that filter, counterbalancing threat with safe experiences. Without doing that, efforts to improve things would have been undermined by ongoing physiological threat processes.

The run-up period

In the months and years prior to illness onset or worsening, your body may have been working hard to restore balance in the face of disruptors you didn't register (e.g. work stress, minor illnesses, excessive drinking or sugar intake). Your body has a trait that you may well relate to. That is the tendency to get on with mounting difficulties quietly and independently until it has to really scream for help. You hear that scream in physical symptoms and mood changes. It wasn't that everything was fine up until the point of screaming, you just hadn't been alerted sufficiently. When you can recognize what commonly contributes to the accelerated build-up of allostatic load, you can make some updates to help your body out.

See if you recognize any of the following.

Normalized high stress and/or life transition(s)

Before Heather fell ill, she was navigating new independence as she completed university and entered the working world. Sure, she found things challenging, but she had been used to that, she told me. She skipped over the period of the pandemic as 'just one of those things' that everyone went through. She told me, if anything, it was a relief to not have to go into the office. When I asked her why, she casually told me how she generally felt a high sense of social anxiety. Again, to her this was nothing of note. It was her everyday experience of life. But this ongoing social anxiety had been adding to her allostatic load on a daily basis. Heather thought that none of this was *particularly* stressful because other people didn't find them stressful.

This is one of several ways I see people normalize experiences that are negatively affecting them psychologically and physically. Other normalization logics are things like being used to the stress or having 'gone through worse'. For some, stress is even exciting, so it is assumed that it can't physically affect you. As explained on page 44, the physical experience of stress happens when your body has to activate to meet demands. Repeated activation, whether excitement-induced or not, can be physically depleting over time.

A tendency to cope through busyness

Feeling like you are doing something is a natural comfort during difficult times. When there are problems, finding a solution is rewarding in the brain. Sometimes the act of looking for solutions can feel good (or productive) but it can leave you constantly searching without adequate rest or reprieve, building allostatic load. This is in part due to your dopamine system, which drives you to act. These dopaminergic systems are consistently stimulated in a society that values progress and attainment. At every turn it is socially reinforced that you should busy yourself to meet expectations or find fulfilment. Just *being*, can be threatening on a psychological and biological (psychobiological) level. Instead, your dopamine systems and SNS keep you activated and busy, contributing to long-term depletion without adequate opportunities for equalizing.

Seeing emotions as things to be fixed

People are generally taught to process difficult emotions by *fixing* them and getting rid of the emotional discomfort. This teaches the brain that being with negative emotions and experiencing them is threatening.[14] When you go through hard experiences that naturally give rise to difficult emotions that can't be fixed (e.g. break-ups, losing your job, getting ill) the brain elicits the threat response, which can add to allostatic load.[15] When I asked Heather in our early sessions how she dealt with difficult feelings, her forehead creased as she considered. 'I don't think I really do.'

Experiences of being unheard or on your own

When I shared with my therapist what I was struggling with and what I wanted help with, it was met with silence. Silence followed by a line of questioning that made me feel that the words I was saying were not recognized or perhaps valid. When Heather was held back from school, no one explicitly recognized how this made her feel othered and fragile. Going unheard can make you feel completely isolated and disconnected. Decades of research have shown just how physiologically threatening this is, causing huge disruption to your regulatory systems.[16,17]

Experiencing dismissal in the healthcare system, relationship conflicts, workplace bullying and ostracism are common experiences of being unheard that feature in the run-up to illness.

Pushing your body through sickness

It is societally encouraged to keep going even when you are ill. From adverts for medications that allow you to keep getting things done, to workplaces with strict rules about absence for illness, the expectation is that you 'push on'. In the run-up to illness/illness worsening, there may be lots of instances where this expectation saw you deny yourself time off when you needed it, or going back to work sooner than your body was ready to. In fact, remaining active until forced to rest is a predictor of burnout and health issues becoming persistent.[18,19,20]

For Heather, recognizing all that she and her body had been contending with and expecting of themselves was a relief. It also meant we could pinpoint certain things like social anxiety and emotional coping to reduce ongoing stress, that were likely continuing to tax her systems. This recognition cultivated two important things: compassion for herself and her body, and hope for the, as yet, unexplored avenues to help her body rebalance.

Triggering phase

The triggering phase is the period right before or just as you experience the start or sharp increase of symptoms. This can be the point that people fixate on, with a sense that without this specific event or action everything would have remained on an equilibrium, driving self-blame and regret: 'If only I didn't take on that extra project!' When injuries happen out of the blue or because of accidents, it can feel especially unfair and hard to move on. These feelings create more threat and depletion in the body, making it harder to navigate challenges and feel a sense of hope.

The triggering phase can be misleading as your brain deduces that because this one thing changed (such as diet or sleep pattern or relationship) that is the one thing that needs to be targeted to improve things: the magic fix. It is this logic that can see people try diet after diet to try and fix IBS or scouring the internet for miracle cures that have no real evidence base and potentially potent side effects.

For Heather, her brain was stuck at the point of shock in waking up one day with symptoms that never left – and quite understandably. This was a devastating change to her whole life. Her brain fixated at the point where things suddenly changed, concluding that if only she could figure out what had happened, perhaps she could rectify it and get her life back. This meant that every test she'd had, every investigation, still left her with a sense of incompletion because none of them could adequately explain the sudden shift. Only when she saw how multiple things had been accumulating over her life, did she feel a sense of liberation from this fixation. She realized that the trigger could have been anything at any point and didn't need further attention. She was released to start working with where her body was right *now*.

Moving away from a magic fix

'Magic fixes' are the quick, easy solutions you naturally desire when experiencing illness. The pill that can shift pain or mood disturbances. The quick procedure that can stop bladder troubles. The injection or minor surgery that will get you 'back to normal'. Magic fixes are marketed to you in the form of supplements, diets and weird and wonderful protocols that guarantee you transformation. However, you may quickly discover that the magic fixes aren't

Pre-birth & early years
Biopsychosocial influences on health that you have limited control over from birth

Biological	**Psychological**	**Social**
• Genetics	• Personality	• Parental relationships
• Diet	• Experience of emotions	• Schooling
• Immune function	• Cognitive development	• Security at home and with primary care givers
• Presence or absence of disease	• Coping and habit formation	• Friendships

↓

The run-up period
Different biopsychosocial experiences you may experience prior to illness or burnout contributing to allostatic load and bodily dysregulation

Biological	**Psychological**	**Social**
• Illness	• Mood	• Life changes & transitions
• Exposure to pathogens	• Coping behaviours	• Work environment
• Physical fitness	• Emotional style	• Relationships
• Lifestyle factors	• Health behaviours	• Connection/community
	• Headspace	

↓

Triggering event/s
Common biopsychosocial 'triggers' that can set off illness or burnout after culmination of experiences in the run-up period

Biological	**Psychological**	**Social**
• Exposure to pathogens	• Exposure to stress	• Threatening/hostile social experiences
• Accident or injury	• Mental health/trauma	

↓

Health issues start or worsen

Figure 7: Biopsychosocial factors that influence the development of health issues across three phases, adapted from Chalder & Willis.[21]

working. This can make you feel lost and powerless. The promise of that magic fix is compelling. When you are at your most vulnerable, you crave something to rescue you because it is hard to navigate the complexity. Particularly when you are depleted and your PFC is inhibited by the various biological processes of threat mode, making it harder to figure things out. The expectation to 'sort yourself out' can put debilitating pressure on you.

When you stop waiting to find the 'right' path that will solve everything, you free yourself up physically and psychologically. You reduce the physical effects of self-pressure, and you create more opportunities for your brain and body to feel a sense of control and progress. These are important cues of safety that are physically replenishing.

When working with Heather, we made space to fully acknowledge the multidimensionality of health. She granted herself permission to gradually build habits that would improve symptom experiences and reduce anxiety.

Hearing your body when it whispers

Regaining trust in your body means finding ways to start feeling safe and confident in it again. One of the ways you can do that is by improving your skills at observing earlier those small cues where you're able to intervene. This involves building 'interoceptive awareness': awareness of your internal bodily signals, like your heartbeat, thirst, hunger, and other sensory experiences (e.g. pain, heaviness, sore eyes). You do this all the time without any thought.

Take hunger. Some people can detect hunger as soon as they feel a slight emptiness in their stomach, whereas others only detect hunger when the stomach is grumbling loudly and persistently and they are feeling grumpy. Once detected, some may remain acutely aware of the body's hunger, whilst others may 'forget' that they are hungry. The interpretation of hunger can also vastly differ. For some, hunger is a welcome and safe experience – 'Yes! I get to eat!' – and for others a threatening experience – 'Oh no! I've already eaten too much. I'll bloat out.' This often subconscious process has a big impact on the regulation of internal processes that will determine your body's ability to get back to balance (homeostasis). For example, not eating will impact blood sugar levels, and your metabolic processes, which can make you more likely to feel irritable and/or low and binge eat later.

Interoceptive awareness has a direct impact on the functioning of all the regulatory systems. Your immune system is alerted to invaders (pathogens like viruses or bacteria) through interoceptive processes, allowing it to activate appropriate immune responses. Impaired interoception can lead to the immune system detecting invaders too readily or not readily enough. When too readily initiated, the immune response can result in chronic inflammation present in conditions like inflammatory bowel disease, fibromyalgia, rheumatoid arthritis and more. When too slow, it can lead to poor wound healing and inhibit recovery from surgery or other treatments and leave you open to recurrent infections.

Your metabolism and cardiovascular function are closely influenced by your interoceptive awareness too.[22] When this awareness is intact and stable, your body effectively monitors energy usage and anticipates future energy needs. You experience this balance as steady energy levels. Depending on how interoceptive awareness is disrupted, you may have an elevated capacity for exertion leading you to later crash as you've gone beyond your means. Or you might experience heightened responses to physical exertion like exaggerated heart rate or blood pressure changes, potentially contributing to excessive fatigue.

Interoceptive awareness is therefore hugely powerful in shaping biological processes and your experience of your own body. As allostatic load increases, interoceptive awareness is disrupted, making you feel more mistrusting and alarmed by your body. This fuels further dysregulation. The good news is that nurturing interoceptive awareness helps you to build a trusting relationship with your body once more. And as you re-establish trust, you can reduce unwanted and intense physical symptoms.[23] Chapters 5 and 6 will guide you to build your interoceptive awareness skills.

Acknowledging your journey

To help guide you out of the magic fix trap you may be in, try the exercise below. When my clients do this exercise, it can be bittersweet. While they recognize how much they have dealt with and how hard it's been, which can be confronting and difficult, they also gain a sense of recognition of themselves and the compassion they deserve. Do it at a time when you've got space to be gentle with yourself and opportunities to turn towards comfort.

Use the template in Figure 8 to write out the different biological, psychological and social elements and events in your life that may have added to the demands or disruptions to your regulatory systems and nervous system. You can use the core safety needs on page 54 and Figure 7 as a prompt.

Here's an example from my experience:

In my early childhood and adolescence I had lots of urinary tract infections, which may have biologically added to my allostatic load. It may also have contributed psychologically as I have a standout memory of being in agony in a supermarket when young because of my bladder hurting and not having any control.

In the run-up period, I was partying, working a lot and consuming a lot of alcohol. I was going through difficult relationship experiences and the pressure of entering the world of work. This range of biological (alcohol, sleep deprivation, stress), psychological (stress, pressure) and social (relationship difficulties, work pressure) experiences will have added to my allostatic load.

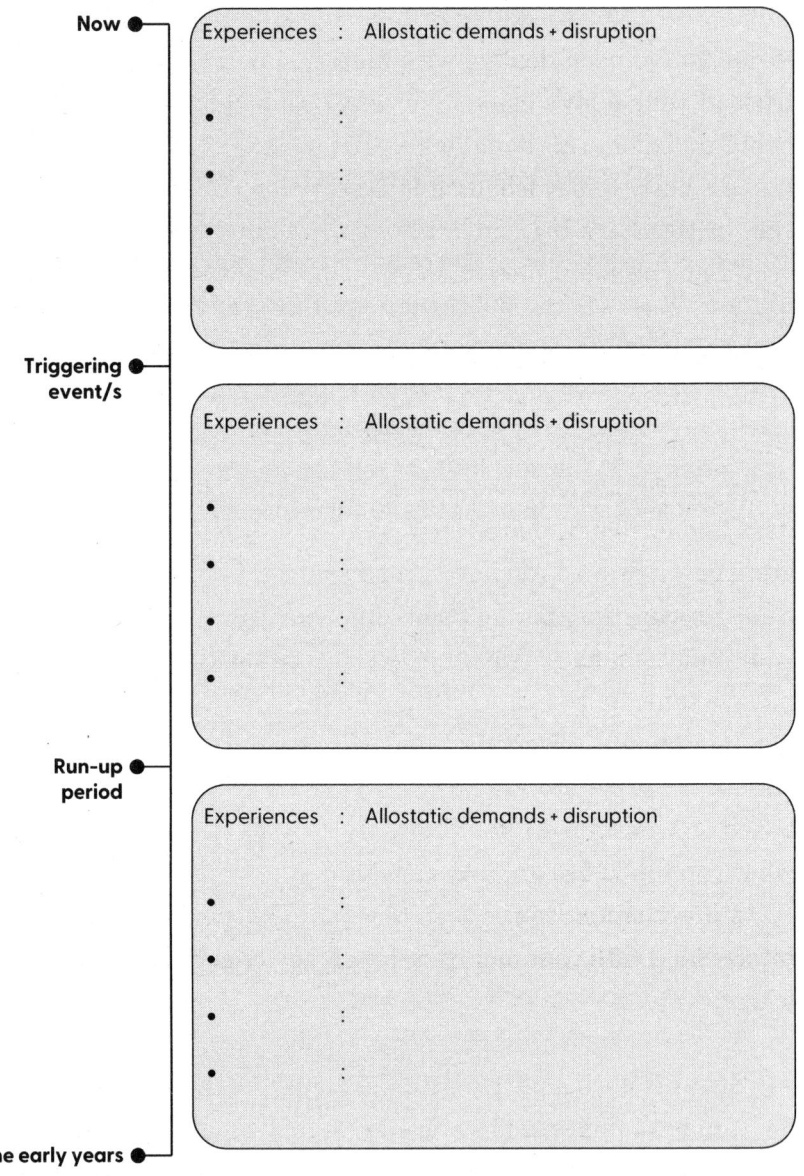

Figure 8: Template for acknowledging your journey activity.

Your body can change: bioplasticity

When you've been dealing with illness, you can lose any sense of trust in your body's capacity to make things better. That idea of being unfixable can hang heavy. The longer your health journey, the less likely it may feel that your body can change for the better. One of Heather's big concerns was that she'd been dealing with symptoms so long, she wondered whether her body was 'too far gone'.

To instil you with hope, I want to introduce you to the concept of 'bioplasticity'.[24] Bioplasticity is when your body adapts and changes to accommodate different experiences. Neuroplasticity is a type of bioplasticity referring to the brain's ability to reorganize itself and form new neural connections throughout life – even creating new neurons. You have already harnessed bioplasticity many times in your life, perhaps without knowing it. As you exercise, your body changes, building better cardiovascular fitness and muscle tone. As you eat more vegetables and less fried food, your gut microbiome diversifies, and your immune system function enhances. These are examples of your body physically updating based on what you do. Your body also physically changes based on what you think, feel and pay attention to.

In this chapter, you've seen how psychological experiences are intertwined with your biological bodily systems. Specifically, you've learnt:

- Stress is itself a physiological event in the body
- You have multiple physiological systems in the body that are impacted by psychological and social experiences (regulatory and nervous systems)
- Your brain and body can turn on 'threat mode' in response to chronic stress and trauma

- There are three key stages of becoming unwell: early years, run-up period and triggering event

Building this knowledge of your biology opens avenues to harness bioplasticity to change your body and improve your health. Avenues that involve working with your psychological and social experiences, that may have previously been unknown or stigmatized, keeping you stuck and lacking choice. Where once you may have felt stumped by your body, now you may see scope for more agency in other places.

I was fortunate to have a solid foundation of understanding the mind–body connection and how my thoughts, emotions and behaviours were affecting my bladder. More than an understanding, I had a support system with a shared understanding that allowed me to explore this connection safely. This exploration changed my relationship with my body from one that was fraught with frustration and feeling betrayed, to one that was gentle and comforting. I stopped storming to the toilet and burying my head in my hands, collapsing into my lap the moment I got that pinching burn sensation. I started calmly checking in with my sense of panic, while remaining where I was, grounding myself, before going to wee.

As that bodily relationship changed and I was able to explore others' experiences of bioplasticity through research and clinical practice, I discovered that there were core principles for befriending your biology to feel better. The first was understanding the biological processes, which we've explored in this chapter. The next principle was the tailoring of an approach to one's own individual experiences and biology. Chapter 2 will arm you with more important knowledge to do just that. The rest of the principles are related to the practices of befriending your biology, which are embedded throughout the rest of the chapters in Section Two.

I hope that the processes leading to ill-health, burnout and trauma are a little demystified and the sense of responsibility and isolation are already a smidgen lighter. To help your body move out of threat and powerlessness, we will continue to work on all of this and more. If it all feels a little overwhelming at this point, don't worry, things will become clearer. See if you can trust that your brain will gradually assimilate things as you go.

CHAPTER 2

Mind–body interactions

What happens in the mind is represented in the body. The inverse is true too. The mind creates a representation of what happens in the body. I've introduced you to the constant conversation happening between your mind (psychology) and body (biology) without your conscious awareness. In Chapter 1, we considered some of the key biological processes that mediate your psychological and social experiences. These are the processes at the heart of the Biopsychosocial Model (Figure 4 on page 20). In this chapter, we'll build on that, further demystifying what some of these mind–body interactions (psychobiological processes) look like in the context of different symptom experiences, including fatigue, pain, gut symptoms and more.

To reduce bodily mistrust, self-blame and a lack of sense of control, it is crucial that you have a good understanding of how mind and body are talking to each other through some of the psychobiological processes depicted in the middle of Figure 9. Just as you can't blame yourself for having an allergic reaction or catching a cold, you can't blame yourself for the automatic defensive processing between mind and body that might worsen or perpetuate illness or mood.

Bioplasticity means that you can help your body to adapt and remodel itself, by working with your biology, psychology and social experiences. When you know what is happening on a biological

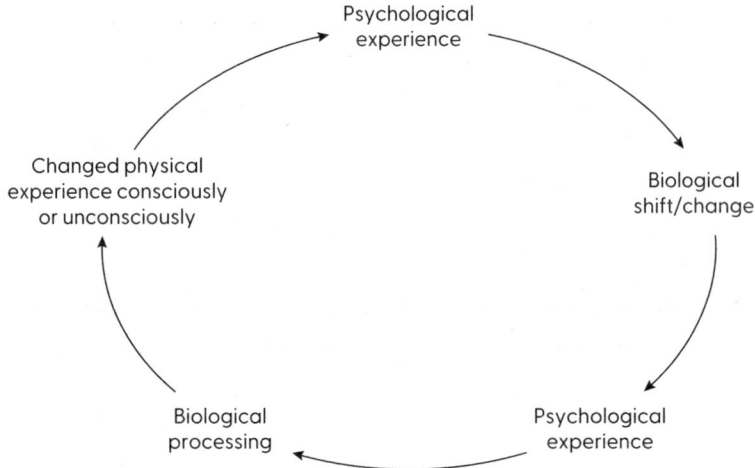

Figure 9: Psychobiological sequences influencing physical health.

level in your body, you can intentionally influence these processes. This chapter will give you clarity about *what* is happening on a biological level in your body and subsequent chapters will provide you with the most well-evidenced strategies for working with these bodily processes.

Anxiety and depression

Moving away from the threat of 'it's all in your head' means changing the assumption that your feelings are your fault. Part of that means acknowledging the impact of the social environments we live in (more in Chapter 7). Another part of that is understanding the biology of psychological experiences and how psychobiological processes can keep difficult mood states going.

Regardless of the cause(s) of depression, there are different elements that can keep it going and exacerbate it – many of which involve psychobiological interactions. A key feature of depression is the suppressed ability to feel pleasure. Research suggests that this experience is underpinned by a biological change to the transmission of the neurotransmitter that is released when you anticipate pleasure or satisfaction, dopamine.[1] Blunted dopamine transmission can dull the reward from doing things and make you feel less motivated to do them. You then change what you do, doing less because it feels like there is no point. The less you do, the less stimulation of the brain's reward centres, the longer depression maintains. Emerging neuroscience research suggests that responding, what can feel counterintuitively, by seeking pleasure or satisfaction and engaging regardless of the dulled feeling, actually stimulates your brain's reward systems.[2] Over time this regulates the dopamine response, and you are again able to access feelings of pleasure and satisfaction. When you know the psychobiology, carrying on despite feelings of 'what's the point?' makes sense. However, if you don't, the biological processes can strongly compel you to back off. We are guided by feelings all the time, so it is intuitive that you would withdraw, and this is not your fault.

People experiencing depression often blame themselves for not looking at things more positively. However, a meta-analysis study combined the findings of twenty-seven studies that explored how processes in the brain change in depression.[3] It found that the brain physically changes how it functions, so that it becomes harder for you to control your thoughts and attention when you are depressed. The same study also found that an area called the default mode network (DMN), which is involved in thoughts about the self, had increased connectivity. This potentially accounts for why, when depressed, the brain circles ruminatively on self-critical and/or defeatist thoughts. This is not a character flaw, but a psychobiological process that needs interrupting with the right guidance.

Similar findings have been shown in the context of anxiety disorders. Brain changes like hyperactivation of the amygdala (threat centre) can keep attention locked into potential threats that further feed feelings of anxiousness.[4] Experiencing ongoing anxiety can also make the ANS and HPA axis more reactive, heightening anxiety.[5]

When you experience a mood state shift, your biology also shifts and that can make it harder for you to find your way out of the emotional experience. Throughout this book, you'll be introduced to well-evidenced approaches that can help to regulate psychology and biology.

Pain, headaches, migraines

The science of pain has advanced a lot. Pain is a sensory process that involves the brain making calculations and predictions about not only whether you should feel pain, but to what degree, for how long and in what way. The brain sifts through information to work out whether you feel stabbing versus burning pain, or a combination, as well as which sensation is dialled up and which sensation is more in the background. Here's how.

Nerves at the site of a pain area may initially be activated because of some irritation or damage. This could be a wound inflicted by something outside the body (e.g. a cut) or it could be an internal wound or irritation (e.g. muscle spasm). This constitutes

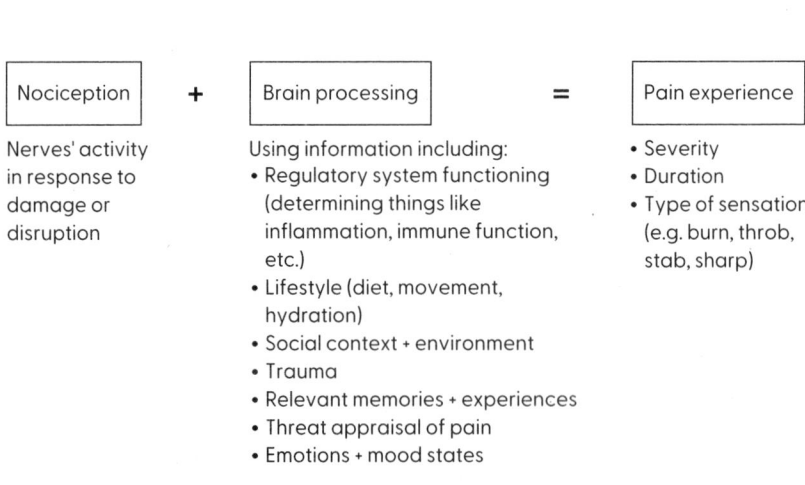

Figure 10: The pain equation, depicting the influence of nociception and psychosocial factors the brain processes.

one part of the pain equation, and this process is called 'nociception'. However, this alone doesn't adequately explain why so many people experience ongoing pain when there are no wounds that should continue activating these nerves. It also doesn't explain why some people can feel little to no pain even when there are significant internal changes to organs or muscles in terms of their health and functioning.

When the nerves transmit messages to the brain, the brain then uses a whole range of information from past and present ('brain processing' in Figure 10) to predict what and how you should feel pain/sensation.

It's like building a fire. The flame to get the fire started is the nociceptive signalling. However, you won't get a roaring hot fire without kindling, logs, enough oxygen and enough heat. These are the various psychosocial factors the brain uses to process pain. Much like a fire, to stop or reduce the 'heat' of pain, you don't need to remove every element contributing to it – just some of the key ones.

Sometimes it is not possible to fully control the elements of a fire just as it may not be possible to fully control pain. Picture a forest fire spurred on by wind that changes direction during a searing hot summer across a sprawling dry forest. Some things you can influence (e.g. dryness), others you can't (e.g. wind). The expectation to completely eradicate your pain can be misplaced and cause too much pressure, actually increasing or maintaining pain. However, it *is* important to have some sense of agency in mitigating pain and its effects.

Areas of the brain that process pain are also areas of the brain that have a role in emotion processing, threat detection, attentional focus, and memory.[6] This physiology can explain why it is so hard to move attention away from sensations of pain, because your brain is set up to prioritize it. It also shows how interrelated pain and emotion are. When you feel difficult emotions, brain regions like the amygdala and anterior cingulate cortex (ACC) activate, potentially increasing the degree of pain your brain calculates. Other research shows that areas of the brain dedicated to helping us understand our social experiences and how socially accepted, rejected or excluded we are overlap with these pain and emotional processing areas (including specific regions of the insular and ACC).[7] A sense of social exclusion and hostility is inherent in 'it's all in your head' messages (page 17). This explains why so many people can experience pain flares in anticipation of socializing, going to the doctor or feeling iced out by their partners.

Layers of pain

Once pain starts, it can become locked in, precisely because of how distressing it is to *be* in pain. Being in pain is a stress to the body's regulatory systems. To unpick this, researchers differentiate 'layers' of pain.

Layer one is the primary layer of the physical pain experience. If I cut my hand enough to require stitches, the sharp sensation and pulling between the parted layers of the skin constitute the primary pain. Layer two is the unpleasantness of pain felt emotionally ('secondary pain affect'). In cutting my hand, I might feel the swell of panic as I see blood dripping and fleshy tissue. I might be filled with fear and urgency to do something quickly. It can be hard to differentiate where layer one ends and layer two begins when feeling pain because they merge together sensorily.

A study used hypnotic suggestion to demonstrate just how much of an impact this secondary layer has on the overall pain experience. Participants in this study all had pain elicited by putting their hands in painfully hot water (safely).[8] They were split into one group that received hypnotic suggestion to 'feel the pain . . . but at the same time, you are not very preoccupied by pain relief', and another group who were induced with negative emotions like sadness or anger. Those who were hypnotically reassured felt significantly less physical pain than their counterparts, who were made to feel anger or sadness. These counterparts also had increased markers of fight or flight arousal (the SNS response, page 42). Working with layer two can therefore interrupt a psychobiological loop that would otherwise keep pain going and/or intensify it. Research has shown that targeting layer two, secondary pain affect, has the power to reduce pain by as much as 50%.[9]

When pain protection makes pain more likely

Pain should be a warning signal so that you can sense injury and respond, but in chronic pain the brain can treat pain like a habit because repeated pain experiences change the wiring of the brain and signalling of nerves. 'Central sensitization' is one way this learning happens, turning the volume up on pain (or potential pain) signals. Over time, the brain can store pain in the same networks used for memories and emotions.[10] This system is evolutionarily intended to help you avoid pain through a good memory of what causes pain, but the processes become dysregulated which means you keep feeling pain instead.

Another way that the biological drive to avoid pain can end up maintaining or worsening it, is through 'pain behaviours'. As your brain learns what hurts, it makes associations of what to do or avoid doing to reduce pain. For example, after a back injury, you may associate bending down, walking upstairs or even showering as 'things to be careful with' or possibly avoid. A highly protective brain (and sensitized nervous system) may mean that you continue to approach these activities with caution or avoid them even when the injury is healed. Pain behaviours can cause the deconditioning of muscles because they prevent you from activity that builds or maintains muscle. Pain behaviours can also increase bodily tension. Deconditioning and tension both contribute to physical pain experiences directly as well as by sending more messages to your brain to be vigilant, thereby turning up the volume on pain sensations.

To help you cope with the distress of pain, your brain can automatically and subconsciously push away pain-related thoughts and feelings. Temporarily this can be helpful, but long term it contributes to more allostatic load (chronic stress), which heightens sensitivity to pain, keeping it going.[11] On the other hand, constantly thinking about pain and what might alleviate it can keep the brain locked into pain.[12] Finding the optimum middle ground to interrupt these psychobiological loops is tricky and involves the principles of interoceptive awareness (page 61). The following chapters will guide you.

Headaches and migraines

Headaches and migraines are affected by these psychobiological pain processes in addition to other interplays between psychology and biology that serve to keep headaches and migraines recurring and/or worsening.

Headaches happen because of a change of blood flow, nerve activity and muscle tension in the head or the neck. These things can also cause migraines. There are additional factors that can play a role in migraines, including abnormal brain activity affecting blood vessels (making them contract or widen), the release of particular neurotransmitters like serotonin and calcitonin gene-related peptide, which can create inflammation and increased sensitivity to sensory stimuli. Because of this and the fact that the neurological changes in migraines are more widespread than headaches, migraines can come with lots of extra symptoms like nausea, change to vision and debilitating pain.

Many things you do impact blood flow, nerve activity, muscle tension, blood vessel activity and the release of neurotransmitters like serotonin. Some of these things will have an acute impact and some will stack up to have an impact later. This makes things pretty tricky for headache and migraine sufferers because it is rarely as simple as 'do this, don't do that'.

Let's take running as an example. Going for a jog could bring on a headache or migraine immediately or soon after because it can impact hydration, blood sugar and tension in the muscles in the neck, head and shoulders, as well as rapidly increasing blood flow to the brain. And yet, regularly jogging can also prevent headaches and migraines long term because it improves cardiovascular health (good for blood vessel health and blood pressure), regulates the release of neurotransmitters with endorphins being released upon exercising and promotes better sleep and mood – all of which can reduce the severity and impact of migraines. Managing hydration and nourishment during exercise is not quite so simple in practice. It takes planning, checking in with your body and balancing. That requires mental capacity for decision-making, which is often depleted in modern-day life, especially so when you've experienced lots of pain or impairment from headaches or migraines. The decision-making process itself can make a migraine more likely.

When you make a decision, a neurotransmitter called glutamate is produced. The more decisions you make, the more glutamate builds up in the brain until it is cleared away, usually through sleep. It plays a crucial role in brain signalling, and excessive levels of glutamate can contribute to the onset of migraines.[13] Glutamate activates neurons (nerves) and when it activates neurons in certain brain pathways, it can cause the dilation of blood vessels (one of the underlying processes of migraines) and can trigger the release of pain-inducing chemicals. You can see how difficult it is to sidestep these psychobiological loops. The good news is knowing this biology can help you to work with it to do just that (more in Chapter 4 on how).

Sleep issues, fatigue & brain fog

Everyone can relate to feeling tired. It is an inevitable experience of life, related to how much sleep you get, how much you are doing, as well as your physical and mental exertion. Whilst tiredness is mostly short term, with a clear cause and effect, generally remedied by sleep, fatigue is the opposite. Fatigue is a persistent experience of tiredness or exhaustion that isn't resolved by sleep or rest. People can experience fatigue as a secondary symptom to another health condition like depression, cancer or sleep disorders, or it can be a primary symptom, such as in chronic fatigue syndrome (CFS), also referred to interchangeably as myalgic encephalomyelitis (ME). ME and CFS are generally viewed as different parts of the spectrum of the same illness, although views vary on this.

Insomnia & interrupted sleep

Sleep is a basic need that has an impact on all aspects of health from basic digestion to mental functioning. A little sleep deprivation may make you a bit less patient or a little more melancholic, but ongoing sleep deprivation can significantly change how you feel and see things. Needing sleep and being unable to sleep can feel desperately scary.

Sleep loss impairs the communication between certain brain networks that are responsible for regulating emotions. The top, front part of the brain that is generally in control of organizing thoughts and decision-making (the prefrontal control networks) starts to have a patchy signal with the area of the brain (in the centre, middle) that produces and processes emotions, the limbic system.[14,15] Usually, the top part would communicate down to the middle part to fine-tune the activity going on there. Where sleep loss impedes this communication, the 'emotional part' of the brain may distort neutral or positive events. With this, emotions can feel much bigger and less controllable. Studies also show that with sleep loss, people tend to feel the need to withdraw more, with a diminished ability to navigate social situations.[16] Sleep disturbances can therefore go round in a hapless loop, altering mood, making life more difficult to navigate, creating more worry and stress, further preventing sleep.

There are lots of biological processes that can make it harder to get to sleep. For some, genetics play a role, with genes affecting sleep regulation and internal body clocks (circadian rhythms). For others, the experience of health issues can make it harder to sleep physically due to pain, discomfort, difficulties breathing or reflux. Medications can also interfere with sleep, as can ingested stimulants like coffee or alcohol.

These biological processes will affect your psychological experience of bedtime, likely making it more pressured or stressful. Stress and anxiety can inhibit your ability to go to sleep and stay asleep, as can other mood disorders like depression because of changes to your neurochemistry and autonomic functioning. The less sleep, the more fear of the negative physical and psychological impacts of sleep deprivation and so the loop goes round. This can build a pressure to sleep.

Pressure to sleep

Intuitively it can feel like you have to make up for lost sleep. This is a concept called 'sleep debt'. Although not outright wrong, the simplicity of it is misleading and it can mean you nervously count down hours of available sleep ('clock watching'). Say, over the last week, you only got four hours' sleep per night because of the baby or feeling unwell or work or maybe all three and you're worrying about how on earth you are going to add in twenty-eight hours of missed sleep. This is not conducive to sleep. It is also not necessary. It overlooks something called 'sleep homeostasis', which is the biological processes that allow the body to flexibly regulate sleep based on how much you need.[17] This need is determined by more than the hours you have slept. Instead, sleep homeostasis takes into account the quality and structure of your sleep. A study by a research professor of sleep and performance and his colleagues found that after chronic sleep restriction, participants did not need to sleep an extra hour for every hour they had lost. Instead, they spent a greater proportion of their recovery sleep in slow-wave sleep, demonstrating that the body prioritizes specific sleep stages based on need. More on this and how to utilize the principles of sleep homeostasis in Chapter 4.

The push and pull of fatigue

There are two common responses to fatigue in the first weeks or months of experiencing it: to try and push through and maintain life at the usual pace or to back off and try and rest enough to replenish the body. Both are understandable and yet both can cause bodily dysregulation. Those who try to push themselves end up crashing with exhaustion as their body doesn't physically have the resource to continue. Those who have been trying to rest fatigue away can feel frustrated with slow (or no) progress and become fearful of activity.

The most confusing thing about fatigue is that it feels like extreme tiredness, so everything you have experienced before fatigue tells you it should go away if only you rest up. Brain imaging studies show that people with chronic fatigue undergo changes in the brain and nervous system in response to the prospect and experience of being physically active.[18,19] The experience of fatigue causes the brain to miscalculate how much effort movement will take, which then ends up increasing how much fatigue individuals feel and how stressful the prospect of certain activities are.[20] These brain miscalculations perpetuate fatigue because too much resting and withdrawal contributes to fatigue. The body gets deconditioned, the cardiovascular, metabolic and nervous systems become less 'flexible', meaning that when you do exert yourself physically or mentally, it creates much more of a splash and all of the internal systems are out of practice in mopping it up. But as we've considered, pushing hard is just as unhelpful as it causes various regulatory systems to work beyond their means, leading to exhaustion and potentially additional symptoms like aches and pains.

Beyond sleep and activity in chronic and post-viral fatigue

CFS/ME is not a sleep disorder, although sleep is likely to be heavily affected. Research demonstrates complex biological processes contribute to the illness including neurological, immune and metabolic dysfunction.[21] There also appear to be many subpopulations under the umbrella of CFS/ME, without one unified underlying cause, making it hard for patients to work out their best course of care. Persistent fatigue has historically (and presently) been met with medical scepticism and often viewed as a 'mental health condition'. Just prior to the publication of this book, a landmark study of over 15,000 people with ME/CFS demonstrated the significant role of epigenetics (environmental activation of genes) in the triggering of the condition.[22] This not only dispels medical stigma but demonstrates the potential role of psychobiological processes in disease onset.

The COVID-19 virus has helped to significantly update the research and understanding of the biological processes that can contribute to fatigue after a viral infection.[23] Such research has demonstrated that the behaviour of cells is altered in those experiencing post-viral and chronic fatigue. The powerhouses of cells are called mitochondria and they produce the energy a cell needs to perform its function properly. Some studies of patients with persistent fatigue demonstrate that the mitochondria do not function as they should, reducing cellular energy production, which means the body's cells cannot meet the demands for energy. This metabolic dysfunction can also result in changes to the immune system, with increased inflammation and immune exhaustion. When the body is depleted in this way, there is more of a risk of catching infections and impeding the ability to recover quickly.

ANS dysregulation is commonly seen in post-viral fatigue patients, resulting in changes to blood pressure and heart rate.[24] As you've seen, the ANS is one of the key superhighways between mind and body. Experiencing elevated heart rate and blood pressure feels physically and psychologically unsafe, sending messages to your brain that there is something wrong. It is hard for the brain to disregard this information, leading to lots of thinking. Many of these thoughts can generate more fear and worry, creating further snowballing psychobiological loops.

Brain fog

'Brain fog' is a term for reduced mental clarity and agility, making it hard to hold things in mind, remember and focus. People describe it like mentally wading through mud with thought feeling slow and 'foggy'. Brain scan studies on patients with chronic and post-viral fatigue who also reported brain fog, have shown elevated levels of inflammation in the brain and nervous system.[25,26] This is found particularly in brain regions dedicated to thinking (cognitive processing) and autonomic regulation (linked with fight, flight or freeze processes). Disruptions in the connectivity between brain regions responsible for attention, memory and decision-making have also been observed, which would explain why it can feel so hard to harness your concentration and work things out.

Brain fog can reduce your confidence in your ability to think, remember and problem-solve. You might avoid situations that require concentration like particular work tasks or meeting new people where you fear judgement for slowed thinking. Unfortunately, this can weaken pathways in your brain involved in harnessing attention and short-term memory, potentially keeping brain fog going.[27,28]

Pushing your brain when you have brain fog is not the answer either. If you've ever lost grasp of a word mid-sentence, you may be familiar with the stand-off you have with your brain as you try to find it. The gap between you thinking and speaking widens, disrupting the flow of thought. This is a similar process to what happens when you try to push through brain fog. Your brain needs a lot of energy to keep focus especially when mentally fatigued. When you keep pushing, you increase your brain's demands of blood sugar (glucose) and oxygen – often beyond what your body can easily supply. This can worsen brain fog. When you try to keep focus you rely heavily on the PFC to direct attention and figure out your thoughts. Studies show that overworking the PFC can deplete brain chemicals (neurotransmitters) that support focus, making it progressively harder to think with clarity.[29] Once again, the answer to working with your body is finding the middle ground to regulation.

Recurrent or chronic infections & autoimmunity

The immune system is the body's defence against invaders (pathogens like bacteria or viruses) that can make you sick or disrupt your body's status quo. It does this by identifying the invaders and then targeting them to break down and eject them. The immune system is spread throughout the body. It is in your skin and membranes that produce mucus (like your nose or bowels). Other key parts of your immune system are:

- **Bone marrow** – produces white blood cells that search for pathogens
- **Lymphatic system and lymph nodes** – a network of vessels carrying immune cells and immune filtering structures

- **Spleen** – filters blood to remove damaged cells and produces and activates immune cells.

Your immune system can have a general first line of defence to any invader that appears unfamiliar, and it can have a more targeted 'adaptive immunity'. This is where it learns to recognize specific invaders to make future attacks on them more efficient. This is what happens when you get vaccinations: a little of the virus is introduced so your immune system can power up a strong defence when it comes across it in the future.

In a healthy body when everything is balanced and the regulatory systems are in good health, the immune response runs smoothly. You can feel your immune system in action when you get a cold. Things we think of as 'cold symptoms' like a runny nose, burning throat and congestion are not the cold virus itself, but your immune system responding to fight off the virus. When there are imbalances (biological or psychological) this can affect how the immune system functions.

Inflammatory processes

A seminal study in the Nineties demonstrated that being chronically stressed disrupts your immune system's ability to physically heal. This was starkly illustrated in the additional 9 days it took for the wounds of stressed carers to heal versus their non-stressed counterparts.[30] The disruption to the immune system processes is due to the continued activation of the HPA axis (page 42), keeping the production of stress hormones like cortisol going. The ongoing drip of these hormones suppresses the production of immune cells necessary to fight off invaders and so it becomes harder for your body to fight off infections. Dysregulation in the HPA axis leads to dysregulation in the inflammatory response.

The overactivity of the SNS and underactivity of the PNS also dysregulates the inflammatory response. A little bit of inflammation helps the body fight infections and allows skin tissue to heal. When you cut yourself and a scab appears, this is the immune inflammatory response in action. The inflammatory response allows more blood containing immune cells to flow to the wound site to fight infection and start to repair the tissue. As part of this inflammatory process, platelets in the blood start to clot (scab) to stop the bleeding and protect the wound while the skin tissue underneath is being repaired. Under that scab, inflammation continues to clean out debris and fight infection.

If there is too little inflammation, wound healing is slowed. However, if there is too much inflammation it can lead to the damage of healthy tissues (like skin, muscle or organs) as there is continuous immune cell activity that can degrade collagen, produce scar tissue or break down healthy skin, muscle or organ tissue, as happens in illnesses like inflammatory bowel disease, lupus, rheumatoid arthritis and multiple sclerosis. Shared experiences across inflammatory conditions include pain, changes in energy level and disruption to usual bodily functioning, making days more unpredictable and harder. This experience itself is stressful, impacting what you are able to do and how you feel about doing/not doing it. Herein lies another psychobiological loop: the dysregulated immune system creates physical experiences that are emotionally and behaviourally dysregulating. The results of which can further dysregulate the immune response

'Sickness behaviour'

When you are depleted and your immune system is working overtime, you have a hardwired biological response called 'sickness behaviour'.[31] Sickness behaviour covers a range of automatic behavioural and physiological responses to infection, as the immune cells act on regions of the brain to produce behavioural changes. These include:

- Social withdrawal
- Depressed mood and apathy
- Fatigue, lethargy and sleep disturbances
- Increased sensitivity to pain.

Evolutionarily these behaviours conserved energy, which could then be redirected towards the immune response. It also ensured survival, by reducing potential vulnerability when not adequately resourced to fight or flee.

However, in modern times, withdrawing can do you a disservice. It stops the mood-buffering effects of feeling connected (more on this later). Reduced appetite and lethargy mean you are less likely to engage in important care-taking behaviours for yourself, like making nutritious foods or prioritizing hydration. Low mood triggered by illness can cause further downward mood spirals that are hard to emerge from, giving rise to more difficult thoughts and feelings. The increased sensitivity to pain can also start interacting with pain processes described earlier, exacerbating symptoms and making them harder to deal with.

Whatever the initial cause(s), the experience of repeated infections or symptoms of autoimmune diseases create more stress and imbalance in the regulatory systems. This dysregulation (and disruption of immune functioning) can be perpetuated by the emotional impact of sickness and sickness behaviours. As is the theme running across the other sections considered so far, healing is about finding the right balance.

Gut issues

Gut issues can be completely life-changing. Angry heartburn, reflux, painful cramps, urgent sprints to the toilet or stubborn straining stints, all have the ability to affect your relationship with basic functions like eating and defecating. This can make you feel different to others. Having to organize life around toilet access or no longer being able to eat your favourite foods, dealing with pain or stigmatized symptoms when socializing all take their toll. Where you witness others go to the pub casually, you judiciously select a non-alcoholic or bubble-free option. You may believe that these things are purely unfortunate consequences of having gut issues. And to some extent they are. These ways of coping come after the symptoms start and yet they also may play a significant role in the psychobiological feedback loops that keep symptoms going.

From the mouth to the anus, everything in the digestive system is working to break down food, absorb nutrients or expel waste. This is done by the release of chemicals to break down food in your saliva and stomach, through muscle contractions across the gut (in particular the colon) and the production of mucus to facilitate the movement of food and waste. When things go wrong in the gut, people intuitively explore the impact of food. The assumption being that something problematic has made contact and upset things. Yet this doesn't explain why (outside of food intolerances, allergies and conditions like coeliac disease) people often don't have consistent reactions to specific foods. Or why in inflammatory bowel disease, people continue to get intense cramps or pain when the condition is otherwise managed by medications.

Gut behaviour

Having gut symptoms may incite you to change your diet and eating patterns, skipping food altogether at times. You may change your activities and exercise routines, toileting rituals (straining, pre-emptive emptying, being on the lookout for the toilet) and use medications like laxatives or ones that slow or stop bowel movements. Some of this may be necessary, however all these reactions also end up changing how the gut works and can potentially contribute to further bowel dysregulation.

Meal-skipping makes sense if you're in pain or nauseous. And yet, the gut is a creature of habit much like a dog that stares at you pointedly in the evening when it is 'treat time'. Or starts misbehaving when it hasn't been on its usual walk with an opportunity to expel its energy. The gut requires regularity of certain things for muscle contractions to remain regular and coordinated. Being fed consistently is one of them. Sleep and activity patterns are another. If you start changing how you eat in response to symptoms, it can confuse the gut further. As the gut gets more confused, the gut contractions (peristalsis) become more uncoordinated. This can perpetuate cramping, pain and/or change in stools. It can also change how able the stomach is to break down food. For example, if you end up eating larger meals later in the day because you haven't eaten during the day for fear of symptoms, it can make it harder for digestion. Not only will you soon be lying horizontally in bed, meaning gravity is not aiding the process of digestion, but your body is powering down and slowing digestive processes and affecting how your gut feels.

Feelings about your gut create feelings in the gut

I've had consultations with patients in floods of tears as they describe the devastation of gut symptoms. People have altered major life decisions because of gut issues. Some have withdrawn from university or have left their job. These decisions aren't made lightly and they have their own far-reaching impacts on health and life trajectories. The fear of pain, the shame of bowel symptoms or the erosion of self-confidence can mean people feel they have little choice.

The emotional reactions to symptoms are central to addressing symptoms. Emotional reactions to gut symptoms have an impact on biological processes in the gut. Fascinating research has demonstrated a link between the tendency to push down feelings and the health of the bacteria and microorganisms living in the gut, called the gut microbiome. The gut microbiome has a huge impact on gut function as well as many other body functions including the immune system and organs like the bladder. A Harvard study followed nurses during a six-month period exploring the relationship between emotional experiences and the gut. Emotional suppression reduced the diversity of the gut microbiome.[32] This is a wonderful illustration of how your relationships with your feelings can shape your physiology.

Emotional experiences, thoughts and perceptions are inextricably linked with gut function via something called the gut–brain axis. This is the two-way communication superhighway that feeds nerve signals to and from the gut. Your enteric nervous system resides in the gut. This is a sub-branch of your nervous system that is made up of 100 million neurons, 90% of which are dedicated to sending messages *to* the brain independently, unlike most other organ systems which instead are generally working to receive and act upon messages *from* the brain. This may well be why language reflects the close relationship between the gut and feelings: gut instinct, gut feeling, butterflies in your stomach, stomach drop. Emotions are often most physically felt in your gut.

The difficulty is that you get a lot of information from the gut. And if your brain is primed to perceive sensations in the gut as a threat, as it often is due to uncomfortable symptoms, this communication can get loud. The increase in volume is underpinned by increased activity in nerve cells, that feed more information back to the brain, making you feel even more sensation in the gut. This gives more alarming data to the brain, which can then turn up the volume of the nerve signals in a vicious cycle.[33] The term given to this process of increased productivity of the nerves in the gut is 'visceral hypersensitivity' and affects approximately 30–40% of those with irritable bowel syndrome.[34]

As you may imagine, the more we feel, the more our brain pays attention. The more thoughts it generates about what is going on, the more we feel the need to react. Together, these changes continue to alter the biology of the gut, often keeping it stuck in cycles that we are desperate to escape.

Bladder & pelvic problems

The media and social discourse about gut health and bowel function has increased over the years, reducing the taboo around them. However, stigma around bladder and pelvic symptoms remains. Those who have symptoms like needing to pee more frequently or urgently, pain or discomfort in the bladder, urethra, vulva, vagina or surrounding pelvic regions and urinary retention, tend to feel these things are shameful or embarrassing.[35]

These are symptoms that instinctively people feel the need to keep hidden. Part of this may be because pelvic and bladder issues can feel inextricably linked with sex and genitals. Sometimes it can be hard to precisely pinpoint sensations which can create confusion and awkward encounters with doctors and nurses. So strong are these uncomfortable feelings towards these symptoms that one American survey found that as many as 71% of women had not discussed their experience of vaginal discomfort with their doctor.[36]

Shame perpetuates and worsens pelvic pain

Patients with pelvic and bladder issues often report being frowned at or interrogated, because their symptoms seem unusual to the practitioner and because patients struggle to articulate their symptoms due to embarrassment.[37] People clam up or try and play down symptoms when they are made to feel like this. The unfortunate result is that they are less likely to get access to the investigations and care they need.

Shame can also directly affect pain and pelvic symptoms.[38] An interesting illustration of this comes from one study of 974 college women, exploring the experiences of pain in penetrative sex for young women. Those who felt higher guilt around sex had more pain during intercourse.[39] Multiple mind–body (psychobiological) pathways could explain this shame/pain relationship in the pelvic region. One likely culprit is the pelvic floor. The muscles of the pelvic floor span the area between your pubic bone at the front of your pelvis, the tailbone at the back and the sides of your hips. They create a hammock-like structure at the base of your pelvis and support the bladder, intestines and, in women, the uterus and vagina, keeping everything in place, aiding control in the release of urine and faeces, and vaginal functions.

As with many other muscles in the body, psychological stress causes an automatic increase in tension. Shame can create ongoing stress, causing tension in the pelvic floor. This tension can contribute to many symptoms including pain, urinary tract infection-like sensations, bladder and bowel issues and sexual dysfunction.

Shame can also elevate autonomic arousal,[40,41] further changing bladder function.

Brain, bladder and hormones

The more shameful symptoms feel, the more stress you experience from symptoms and the more tension. Tension and stress change how your bladder (and pelvic floor) behaves and what bladder/pelvic sensations you feel.

There are some well-trodden pathways between the brain, bladder and pelvis. They are in constant communication regardless of whether you have symptoms or not. Part of this is to determine whether your bladder is full and whether it is an appropriate time to relieve yourself. Your brain weighs up signals of fullness from nerves in the bladder, and how much access you have to a toilet. There are multiple brain regions involved in this, including the PFC (the director of attentional focus) and the hypothalamus. The PFC is the reason the urge to pee may increase as you put your key in the lock of your door. The PFC has logged you're nearly at your toilet – a safe place to wee – and has given the bladder the go-ahead signals, leaving you hopping about.

The hypothalamus you may remember from Chapter 1, as having a key role in orchestrating the stress response in the HPA axis and ANS. The bladder is innervated by both the SNS (fight or flight) and PNS (rest and digest), both helping muscles in the bladder to contract and relax at appropriate times. The activation of the SNS allows the bladder to fill from the kidneys, while keeping the urethral muscles contracted, so you don't leak. When it is time to wee, the PNS needs to activate so that you can relax enough to release the urine.

The problem is, when you have been feeling stressed about bladder symptoms, it is difficult to relax when it comes time to wee. If you have experienced a high level of pain upon urinating due to urinary tract infections or tissue damage from birth trauma, for example, your body may automatically brace itself for the event. When you brace, the SNS activates creating muscular tension. This dysregulation to the delicate balance of autonomic activity can cause bladder muscle spasms, urinary retention and wider pelvic floor issues.[42,43]

This dysregulation can also mean that nerves in the bladder change how they behave. They can get more reactive, meaning that you experience lots more sensory messages from the bladder.[36] When all is well, the nerve cells should only communicate fullness of the bladder and the presence of pathogens or other irritants. This can alert the brain to activate an immune response where necessary. Like we explored in the gut, nerve cells can upregulate, becoming more reactive to smaller messages. As nerves upregulate, you may feel premature bladder fullness or odd sensations that indicate an infection or irritant even where such things aren't present.

Urological researchers are increasingly interested in the role of 'neurotrophins', which you can think of as power-boosters for nerve cells that make them do more of what they already do. For example, if the job is to raise the alarm, it allows the nerve cell to raise the alarm louder, more quickly or indiscriminately. In people with a range of bladder conditions, a significant amount of neurotrophins have been found in the bladder wall.[44,45] This likely accounts for the upregulation of bladder nerve cells resulting in increased discomfort and hyperactivity of the bladder. Certain neurotrophins can be released in the experience of stress, to help your brain cope. The more you go through stress, the more your brain may release neurotrophins to help you deal with stressors and strengthen connections. The difficulty is that when the physical experience is the stressor, the connections being strengthened are ones that keep these symptoms going.

Just like the bladder (and the gut), the pelvic floor has nerve cells that are susceptible to upregulation and can become overactive. A phenomenon called 'cross organ sensitization' means that nerve cells in one region of the body that are similar in structure and function to those found in another area (often not too far away, like the bladder and pelvis) can mimic transmissions going on in their nerve counterparts. This is one reason why pain can move around or spread.

Nerves are not the only things to change their behaviour when feeling stressed by bladder or pelvic symptoms. As the HPA axis maintains an ongoing stream of stress hormones like cortisol, adrenaline and norepinephrine in response to ongoing stress (potentially arising from the symptoms themselves), this can affect blood flow in the pelvic region. Over time this can in turn alter the muscle tone and function of the pelvic floor, maintaining or worsening symptoms. When you force yourself to pre-emptively go to the toilet, or automatically hyperfocus on what the bladder or pelvic region feels like, you are unknowingly feeding into this evolving psychobiological feedback loop.

Bad periods

If you have a period, you will have your own conceptualization of a 'bad period'. For some, it will entail high levels of debilitating pain, even fainting and nausea. These are not 'normal' experiences and should be investigated extensively, ruling out the possibility of polycystic ovary syndrome (PCOS), endometriosis or adenomyosis. It takes on average seven to nine years for such conditions to be diagnosed, despite many experiencing 'bad periods' from adolescence.[46] As with all conditions, PCOS, endometriosis and adenomyosis benefit from the processes described in this book. However, like any condition, it is also crucial to be biomedically informed with appropriate treatment options.

Bad periods may also describe feeling intense mood swings around the time of menstruation, high anxiety or even body dysmorphia. Understanding what might be behind increased pain and more intense mood disturbances requires an understanding of the impact of hormonal changes across menstruation. The menstrual cycle consists of four stages: the menstrual phase (period), the follicular phase (the body prepares for ovulation), ovulation (an egg is released ready to be fertilized in the right conditions), and luteal phase (in absence of fertilization, this resets the cycle for it to begin again). The menstrual cycle phases are primarily driven by fluctuating hormones, namely oestrogen and progesterone. These hormones act on neurotransmitters in the brain which regulate emotion and behaviour. Oestrogen boosts the production of 'happy chemicals' serotonin, dopamine and endorphins. In the follicular phase, as we get ready to ovulate, there is a rise in oestrogen which often may be accompanied by an improved mood and more energy. This can be a big contrast to menstruation and even the luteal phase, where oestrogen lowers and with that you can feel your mood lower or anxiety intensify.

These hormones impact on your brain–pain circuitry because

they act on certain neurotransmitters and receptors that are involved in pain processing. Oestrogen can increase pain sensitivity, while progesterone tends to have a pain-relieving effect. Hormonal fluctuations can vary the sensitivity to pain. Hormonal fluctuations happen naturally across the cycle stages, but many things including lifestyle, activity patterns, the social environment and your psychological wellbeing can influence how these hormones fluctuate and how the body responds to the fluctuations.[47]

The experience of fluctuating hormones can make you less likely to engage in things that will help to curb the effect of hormone fluctuation. For example, consuming sugary foods and being sedentary (two common inclinations when premenstrual) can boost levels of oestrogen, thereby increasing pain. This does not mean that one day of sugary food consumption and lying on the sofa will make pain worse, but rather developing these habits in response to cycle phases can negatively affect the experiences of the menstrual cycle over time. Like with allostatic load, the effect accumulates. Preliminary research suggests that some people may be more susceptible to physical and psychological symptoms related to hormonal shifts.[48]

People often note that during their menstruation or later luteal phase, they experience more bowel symptoms, having looser stools and more flatulence. This is because the change in oestrogen and progesterone stimulates the release of another hormone, prostaglandin, which triggers contractions that help detach and eject the uterine lining during menstruation. Prostaglandins can also create contractions in the bowels often resulting in looser stools/diarrhoea. It can be hard to tell the difference between menstrual cramps and bowel cramps and this can complicate things further for people with bowel conditions. Prostaglandins are also responsible for the headaches that can come with bad periods.

Dismissing significant women's health issues as 'just hormones' is a common phenomenon. Rhetoric like this feeds into the sense that you are powerless to your biology and that experience of hormonal symptoms *requires* further biomedical treatment to make any difference. That is not to say that biomedical treatment is not important and that recent increased awareness of hormonal replacement therapy (HRT) has benefitted many women dealing with debilitating menopause symptoms.[49] However, going back to that dichotomy that can arise between psychological and biological approaches (page 69), to feel empowered and connected with your body it is also important to recognize the impact of psychological and social experiences. Research shows the more helpless women feel about their menstrual pain, the worse the pain.[50] Other research has also found that feeling anxious and not having stable social support increases the pain experienced in menstrual cycles.[51]

Exercise and physical activity are proven effective analgesics for menstrual symptoms,[52] but the last thing you might feel like doing when in pain is exercise. When I explore this with patients, they may say something along the lines of, 'You don't know how bad it is, I can't move.' Like the psychobiological sickness behaviour processes, all the signals they are getting from their body seem to be telling them to withdraw, pull back and brace. This psychobiological loop can preclude them from feeling physically and emotionally better. Where this happens and it feels preposterous to suggest movement, I emphasize how powerful gentle movement can be and how it has a cumulative effect over time. It is not a case of 'running off' symptoms, but rather creating a stable base of moving safely with your body when symptomatic and not. Gentle body movements get blood flow going, oxygenate areas of the body, increase the heart rate mildly and communicate back up to the modulatory pain circuits in your brain.

Skin & hair issues

The words 'skin' and 'hair' fail to emulate the significance they have to every single one of us. Skin and hair have the power to shape identities, enhance or hinder self-confidence and transform the perception of others. Skin and hair can have cultural significance. For black women, the decision to wear their hair naturally can be weighted in considerations about social stigma and racism. For men who start balding, it can signify the crossing from one life era to another, the implicit communication of an age bracket that you may not identify with.

More than external aesthetics, skin is a fundamental protective barrier between the internal bodily organs, muscles, bones and tissues and the outside world. Without it you'd be left vulnerable to all sorts of infections and harmful substances. It is also a chemical and microbial barrier containing a diverse range of microorganisms and enzymes that maintain skin health and prevent infections. The skin contains numerous sensory receptors that detect touch, pressure, pain, and temperature, allowing the body to respond to environmental changes and potential threats without your conscious awareness.

Skin issues can be inflammatory (eczema and psoriasis), acne-related, allergic reactions (e.g. hives), autoimmune responses (like alopecia and lupus) or cancerous. This is not an exhaustive range – there are many other types of skin issues. The health of your skin is influenced by and influences many of the regulatory systems and branches of the nervous system we have explored, including the immune system, ANS and the gut microbiome. When experiencing skin and hair issues that cause concern and increase self-consciousness, the brain and nerve signals change communication, so that minor or normal physical sensations can feel more intense. This is called somatosensory amplification[53] and is another psychobiological loop. As the person is made more sensorily aware of their skin, it increases worry and stress. This in turn activates the HPA axis and SNS, causing a secretion of stress hormones. In response, glands in the skin react, inflammation increases and the skin's barrier function can become impaired.[54] This can result in further skin issues.

The worry and emotional impact of this can mean that other health behaviours are negatively affected, changing the delicate balance of other bodily systems like the gut microbiome and immune response. Common health behaviours that can maintain or worsen skin issues include skin picking, scratching or touching due to somatosensory amplification, or self-consciousness. Clients of mine experiencing skin issues and alopecia have often felt torn between actions that are necessary to care for their condition and actions that would make them appear more socially acceptable. An example is makeup. This can irritate and inflame acne and other inflammatory skin conditions, and yet it can feel dreadfully exposing and anxiety provoking to go to work without the shield of makeup. What to do for the best? Go into the office under the concealment of makeup and reduce the exacerbating effects of stress? Or allow the skin to breathe unimpeded by makeup but feel terribly anxious and self-conscious? It is a hard decision to make. What can commonly happen is that people swing between the two: lots of concealment (and with that exacerbation of the skin issue) followed by periods of trying to up skin-interventions with medications, tonics and creams. Usually this will come with more solitary time as people feel more self-conscious.

With alopecia, the prospect of losing one's hair can cause a whole host of responses that range from frantic attempts to fix it through to avoidance and resignation. Attempts to fix it may be centred around the appearance or the treatment or both. The difficulty is that urgency and fear that comes with the prospect of hair loss can fuel impulsive decisions to try harsh chemicals or miracle cures on the internet. Many of which can damage the scalp further. Attempts to hide the extent of hair loss with hair products, extensions or tight hairstyles can also end up causing further hair loss due to traction alopecia and hair breakage.

When looking at the intersection between psychology and biological processes in skin and hair issues, as with other physical symptoms, it is important to move away from self-blame. Understanding that negotiating that middle ground to restore balance isn't always straightforward and in the process of negotiating what this looks like, it can feel incredibly vulnerable and difficult. People who manage this find a whole new way of relating to their experience and their skin. The following quote from a participant in a study exploring the role of self-compassion in adjusting to skin conditions is a wonderful illustration of that:

'I just see it [psoriasis] as my body telling me that things aren't right, my systems aren't coping, so when it happens I try to think, "right, what can I do to bring my body back into alignment?"'[55]

Working with your biology & befriending your body

When you are socialized to work with your biology predominantly by outsourcing to medical systems, it can feel impossible to understand how to directly influence your biology yourself using psychology. It is important to clarify that it is not a case of choosing one approach or another. With my patients, my assessment process involves thoroughly ensuring that they have received appropriate medical or physician support, often supporting them to access it where they have not. I have collated some resources and signposting for a range of conditions.* Part of befriending your body means advocating for it to get the support you need. The balancing act is doing this, while not putting too much pressure on yourself.

---

* Signposting and resources available at www.healthpsychologist.co.uk/itsallinyourbody

When I learnt about the role of the nervous system in my bladder and migraine symptoms, it was like a door of hope opened. I could now see an avenue for working with my body rather than expending so much energy hating it and getting angry at it. I shared earlier that I had at one stage banged my head against the wall when having an intense migraine. An illogical action that was purely an expression of intense emotion and desperation. It also reflected how far my attitude to my body was from nourishing and caring for it. It was angry, indignant and violent. When I learnt more about how my body was working, I started to see my body as its own person. One that I needed to coax, so that it could feel better. From this place, when pain started up or my bladder symptoms started twinging, my tone was different:

'Oh dear, what's upsetting you? It's OK, let's see what we can do.'

My escapades to the doctor's were less from a place of, 'Let's sort you out once and for all', and more so, 'Let's see if we can better understand you and help you out a little'.

This attitude shift was utterly transformational. My body seemed to feel less scared in return. Rather than ringing the alarm loudly that something was wrong, it was quieter, more trusting that I was listening to it.

Don't worry if this seems far from where you are. In the coming pages, gradually, we will work on helping you relate to your body in this way too. In fact, at this point, you may like to set a steppingstone goal. Use the exercise below to help you.

Write down your answers to these questions:

- If this chapter has helped you understand a little more about how your mind and body are or have been reacting to each other, jot down what is clearer to you now. Are there ways you have been misunderstanding your body?
- When you experience symptoms (or difficulties more broadly), what is your tone to yourself and/or your body? Describe it as much as you can.

> • What tone or attitude would you like to have when you experience difficulties? Describe in as much detail with examples of phrases or actions. Use the Introduction to help make this into a stepping-stone goal (page 25).

In this chapter you've learnt:

- Some of the underlying biological processes, like brain activity and neurochemical transmission of mood states like anxiety and depression
- How different psychobiological loops can occur as biology meets behaviour, thoughts and feelings
- What a range of different psychobiological loops can look like in common symptom experiences like persistent pain, bowel and bladder issues and fatigue
- How psychobiological loops may keep the body 'triggered' by itself. For example, nociceptive pain signals alerting the brain, which can then sensitize nerves causing more pain.

As we come to the end of Section One, you have digested a lot of science, some of which may make perfect sense to you and clarify things, and some which may have prompted more questions. Perhaps make a note now of how you feel going in to Section Two where we are about to get much more practical. What would you like to get more clarity on or build on? Section One has been about building the foundational knowledge of the mind–body connection, so you can feel confident in the changes you are about to make and clear about how these changes will help you to reach your healing goals. As you go into Section Two, remember, your experiences are never 'all in your head'. Your brain and body automate reactions when in threat mode and need some coaxing. The principle of bioplasticity means that you can gently start to update these bodily defaults.

SECTION TWO

Transforming your experience of symptoms

'I have glimpses of freedom and it's not dependent on my symptoms'
— PATIENT REFLECTING ON THEIR CHANGING
RELATIONSHIP WITH THEIR BODY

How are you feeling now? Do your body and mind feel far too vast and complicated for you ever to truly know, much less influence? Or does it all feel intriguing and like answers are going to materialize as you explore further?

As you work through *It's All In Your Body*, you will likely feel caught between these two sentiments. They are reflective of how your sense of control may fluctuate every day. A distinct feeling of 'I'm going to master this, I'm redoubling all my efforts', giving way to 'what's the point, nothing seems to work?' These underpin the all-or-nothing patterns we tend to fall into as humans.

Let's right now make an intention to find the middle ground. The middle ground is powerful. Instead of grasping for complete certainty and control, try to embrace what feels empowering *now*. Rather than overcommitting to test the extent of your control, try taking things gradually with curiosity and an openness to learn. The benefits of patient openness far outweigh the – often temporary – relief of fast-tracking. *This* is how you make your mind and body feel safe. From that place of safety everything you wish to achieve becomes easier.

In this section I'll share with you the most evidence-based practices to create harmony between mind and body, providing you with a mixture of exercises, reflection points and practical actions. The decades I have spent poring over journal papers, analysing, critiquing and verifying, are now extrapolated in these chapters in a way that will help you take action if you are ready to do so. What brings to life the research concepts measured by questionnaires and biometrics, is the lived experiences of the hundreds of people I've worked with. In the following pages, you will benefit from lessons learnt from the brave vulnerability of others who have shared with me their most harrowing challenges, greatest sadnesses and fears. These are people who have shown up, explored, as you are now, and navigated the messiness that is healing and growth. From their endeavours and my own, I have distilled what it means to work with your biology and stop fighting against your own experience.

By the end of this section, you will know how to:

- Break down, understand and intervene on symptom spirals
- Make small tweaks in what you do for better sleep, energy, digestion and a whole range of physical symptoms
- Feel comfortable with a full spectrum of emotions and how this physically benefits your body
- Feel safe with your own thoughts, interrupting patterns of thinking that trigger threat mode and harness cognitive strategies that improve your physical experience
- Build social safety and advocate for yourself.

All of this will improve the communication issues between mind and body and create a pathway to reclaim your sense of self and belonging. This work isn't easy, and it isn't meant to be. In my opinion, nothing that truly stimulates growth can be plain sailing. Healing is in the drama of the storm and the serenity of it passing.

CHAPTER 3

Interrupting symptom spirals

Earlier, we discussed 'interoceptive awareness': the awareness of your internal bodily signals. Interoceptive awareness is crucial for working out what your body's needs are and meeting them. Your brain pools together data from your physical experience (interoceptive awareness), your psychological experience and your social context in a process called 'multisensory integration'. This multisensory integration is a calculation your brain makes to influence your conscious and subconscious behaviour moment to moment. This process is automated, and you can generally rely on it unless your body is in threat mode due to long-standing physical symptoms, mood difficulties or life stressors. Threat mode disrupts one or multiple inputs to the multisensory integration calculation.[1] Part of befriending your body and working with your biology, involves bringing elements of this multisensory integration from the subconscious to the conscious. Doing so helps you move from a state of automatic threat or disconnection to a sense of safety and empowerment.

In this chapter, you'll be introduced to 'symptom spiral' templates. This will enable you to intentionally break down the multisensory integration process, reducing the automatic reactive psychobiological loops happening under the surface. You'll also be introduced to lots of options for bringing your mind and body back to balance. In the following chapters you'll receive more guidance on how to implement these changes.

Before continuing, you may find it helpful to revisit the goals you created in the Introduction. If you haven't yet created any, you can do so now or directly after this chapter.

The power of observing symptom spirals

Symptom spirals are the rapidly escalating spirals that occur where a symptom triggers a cascade of thoughts, emotions and bodily responses that add layers of physical and emotional suffering. I first met the symptom spiral framework in my early twenties. I was resigned to my fate as I sat on the cat-scratched leather couch at my dad's cottage, greasy-haired, blank-eyed and hopeless. I was signed off work for a few weeks, which was inevitably going to be extended, rendering me incomeless and completely detached from myself and those around me. I was staying with my dad in absence of being able to care for myself and he had invited his partner round to try and pep-talk me. Luckily for me, she was a clinical psychologist specializing in working with people with chronic pain. At that time, she was working in a pain clinic in the NHS.

I don't know if it had been her intention, but she elicited a little from me about what I was going through and perfectly reflected it back to me in a whole new light. My symptoms weren't unknowable. How I felt emotionally and the dark thoughts I was having were entangled with the symptoms and actually influencing them. She had unpicked my symptom spirals. This new vantage point meant that I could now see lots of small, feasible, but potentially hugely transformative, options for changing my reality.

That moment changed things for me. It played a big role in the profession I pursued and, this very moment, in writing these very words. Because in *that* moment, what was going on in my body was not unknowable, after all. That was perhaps the first time I had felt that way in the entire six months or so that I had traversed multiple NHS health departments.

My hope is that introducing the concept of symptom spirals, can do the same for you. The concept originated from a school of psychotherapy, called cognitive behavioural therapy (CBT). It is the most widely used and offered therapy in the NHS in the UK because of the copious amount of research demonstrating its efficacy in improving depression, anxiety, and even post-traumatic stress disorder (PTSD) to the degree that patients are no longer symptomatic.[2] It has been adapted for use in various health conditions, because it creates clarity around communication pathways between mind and body with intuitive avenues for intervention.[3,4]

First introduced to it at my most depleted, it was less than two years later during my studies and research work at King's College London, that I learnt the nuances of the model; how it could be adapted across conditions, the merits of its use in some versus other presentations and the complementary approaches that could enhance its power. I saw how adaptations to the general model based on mind–body science could even improve physical symptoms like pain, bowel issues and fatigue,[5,6,7] altering markers of inflammation and allostatic load.[8]

Although the symptom spiral framework is taken from CBT, there are specific elements in each part of the cycle that are also informed by complementary psychotherapies (acceptance commitment therapy, compassion-focussed therapy, mindfulness, emotional awareness and expression therapy) and the latest mind–body science research. Consider it a framework to make sense of overwhelming or trapping experiences. You'll be guided to interrupt these spirals in the following chapters, utilizing strategies from the most evidence-based psychotherapies and disciplines so that you can tailor what works for your specific difficulties.

Identifying your spirals

When you are in, or anticipate, any situation that is emotionally or physically challenging in some way, your brain and body gear up to automatically respond, often without you having a second (conscious) thought. Think about a time a loved one snapped at you or when you were told you did something wrong. What comes to mind straight away? For some people, it is the emotion, perhaps of irritation or hurt. For others it is the physical feeling. The gut-punch sensation when cross words are levelled at you or the hotness in your body that rises up.

For many of you, what will come to mind first are the many, *many* thoughts about what happened. It doesn't take much for our brains to elicit streams of narration about difficult experiences. The thought stream can often be the first line of defence. Remember the PFC and its role in problem-solving? It tends to be very active as you try and figure out these thoughts and feelings. Beyond making sense of things, it can also spiral when your amygdala (emotion and threat-processing brain region) is over-active. Before you know it, the brain is pumping out a slew of sentiments and projections that make things feel potentially insurmountable. You may go from *that was mean*, to *I must have done something*, to *no I am a complete pushover!* to *I'm going to show them, I'm moving out and they're not going to hear from me until they've grovelled*, all within a few short seconds.

The same thing can happen when you get an unwanted physical sensation. A fairly neutral thought of *'what was that?'* can catapult to *'it's going to get much worse and I'll have to cancel all my plans'*. These thoughts have a big impact on what you do next. The more threatened the thought stream, the potentially bigger or more urgent the response in the brain and body.

Step one of interrupting spirals is to observe them happening and break them down. This is shown in Figure 11.

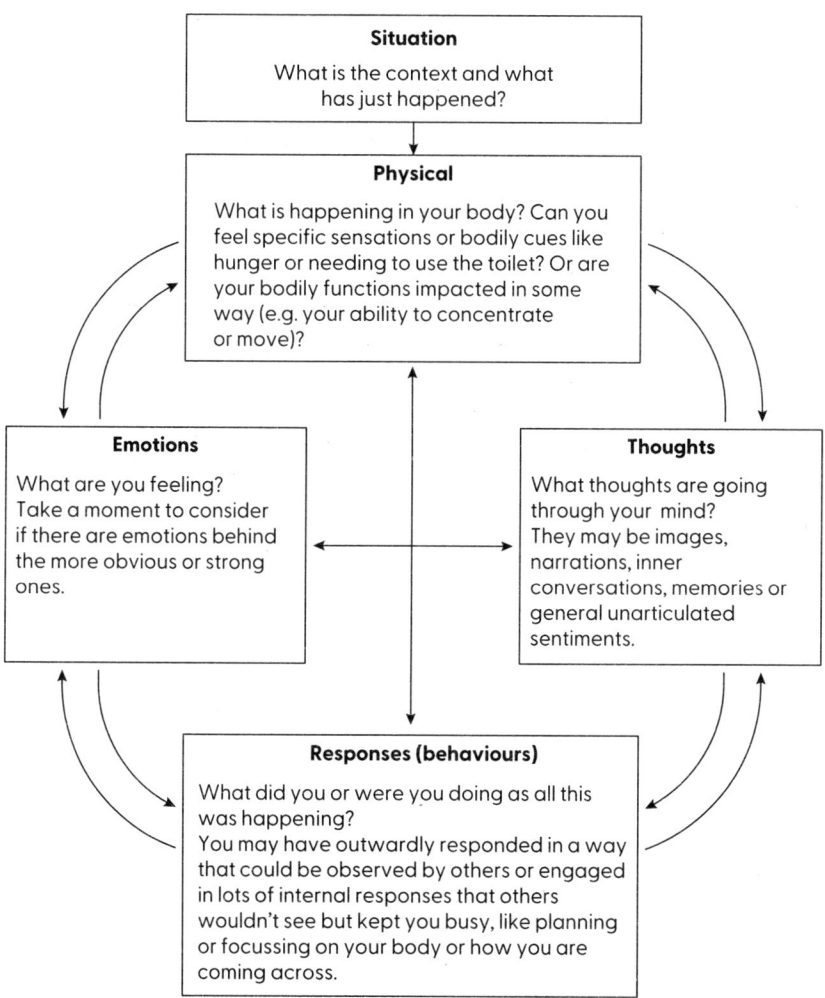

Figure 11: Symptom spiral framework based on Beck's cognitive behavioural model that has since been adapted for physical health conditions.[9]

You can try this now. Pick a situation where you felt distressed in some way. Use Figure 11 to map out each part of the spiral.* Start with whatever part you can recall most easily (thoughts, feelings etc.) then use that to help you recall the other elements. When you've filled everything in, go through it again to see whether, after you acted, more thoughts, feelings or physical experiences unfolded.

Notice how each part of the spiral affects another.

Spiralling

There are two phases that lead to symptom spirals (Figure 12). The first phase involves all the psychobiological processes happening under the surface that create symptoms (as described in previous chapters) and affect the situation you are in. For example, getting cramps because your gut is spasming due to a combination of erratic eating, high stress and a sensitized gut, and these cramps intensifying because of a stressful situation at work.

The second phase is your reaction to the experience of symptoms, which can result in 'symptom spirals' that perpetuate and/or exacerbate symptoms. We can't always influence phase 1, but there is always scope for interrupting phase 2 (symptom spirals).

You can spend hours, days, weeks, months and even years trapped in spiralling cycles without even realizing. What unfolds in one moment, can affect how you relate to things down the line. In previous chapters you were introduced to the psychobiology of threat mode. Where your body is ringing alarm bells, this can change your future thoughts, emotions and even biological responses to similar experiences.

Take this example from one of my darkest periods (Figure 13). When I first started experiencing symptoms that wouldn't ease

---

* You can download a blank version at www.healthpsychologist.co.uk/itsallinyourbody

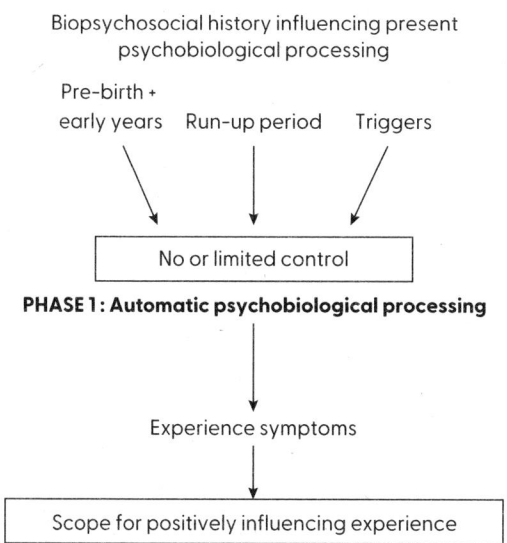

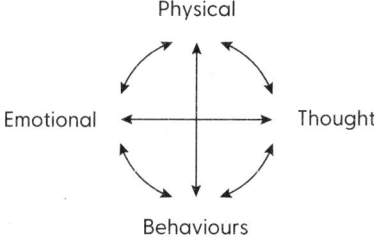

Figure 12: Two phases influencing illness and difficulties with specified scope for personal influence.

with antibiotics, as they had done before, a symptom spiral looked something like Figure 13.

All this worry, fear and hyperfocus interacted with my biology. It was eliciting the biological threat mode and activating my SNS. My amygdala was hijacking my ability to see things from outside of a threat filter affecting my thoughts and emotions. It was also intensifying my physical pain and my actions through the psychobiological processes described in Chapter 2.

This spiral and variations of it, were ingraining patterns of thinking, feeling and responding to my symptoms into my mind and

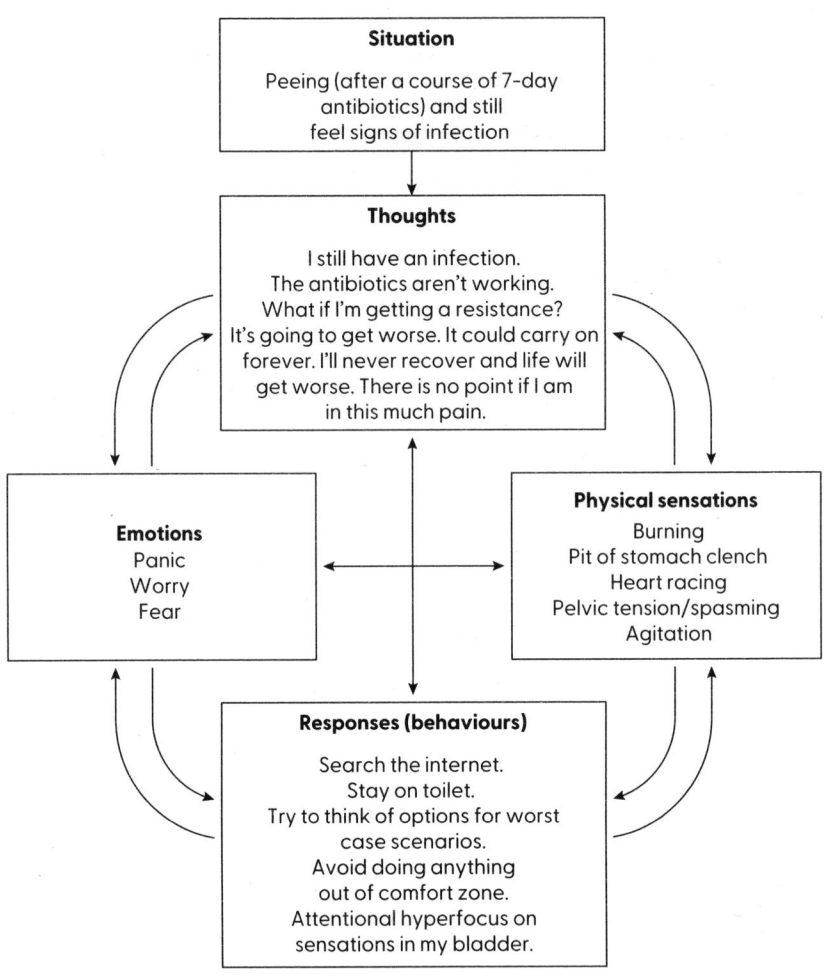

Figure 13: Example of my early symptom spirals.

body. Although the responses might have differed slightly according to new symptoms (e.g. migraines, urgent need to wee or burning bladder pain) or contexts (when on my own, when with others, when at work), my body was learning that I was not safe. My brain was already anticipating the fears before sensations arose. My baseline emotional state was low. My responses and choices were fearful and guarded. This changed how I was experiencing my body and my life in general, feeding more spirals – depressive spirals that saw me questioning the point of life if it was so hard. Anxious spirals that saw me questioning whether people hated me now.

Three months later and a symptom spiral would have looked similar but different (Figure 14). The panic replaced by frustration and resignation, the physical sensations intensified with additional sensations, generalized for longer periods. The thoughts no longer centred around an infection but were consumed by the idea of being stuck with symptoms. The responses were variations of the first intuitive fearful responses: avoid, distract or try to figure out.

Because these spirals are so automatic and threat based, patterns of responding are generally focussed on trying to alleviate the sense of threat in some way. Some responses may be helpful in the short term, but long term can keep the sense of threat and even physical symptoms going. For example, patients of mine with endometrial pain learn to guard their stomachs for reasons they don't always fully understand. It feels comforting in the moment, but it can generalize a sense of vulnerability. Those with bladder issues no longer consider leaving the house without a good knowledge of where toilets are even though this can prime the bladder for action, increasing symptoms. Recoverees from burnout automatically fear job plan changes, their brain anticipating it will mean reduced control over their workstream, creating additional anticipatory anxiety that depletes their capacity further.

The next sections are going to help you get familiar with each element of the symptom spirals so you can better recognize them and understand their influence. This clarity is crucial for you to feel

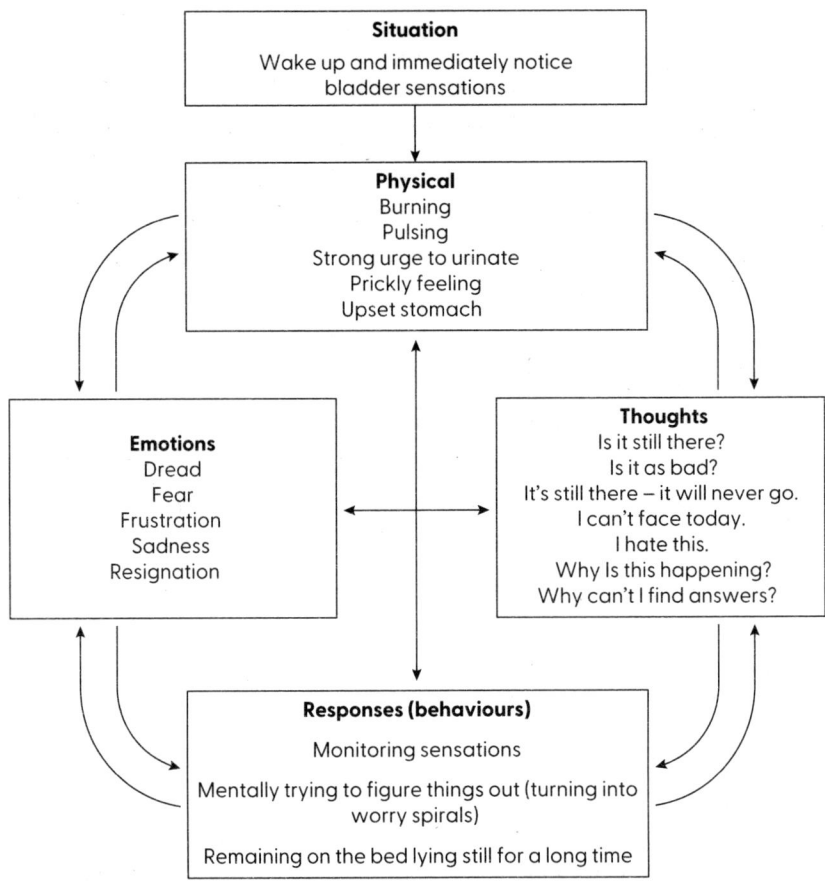

Figure 14: Example of my later symptom spirals.

confident in your own ability to work with your body to make it feel safe again. As this confidence builds, you will feel empowered to make small shifts that make big changes and to let go of strategies that are no longer serving you.

Reacting 'right'

We've discussed the concepts of sickness behaviours: hardwired behavioural responses to physical vulnerability, like infection, evolved to keep you safe and heal. Sickness behaviour directs you to act for short-term relief. Unfortunately, this evolutionary programming can sometimes cause longer-term difficulties in the context of chronic illness, burnout or trauma. The urgency that accompanies the pursuit of short-term relief can also sabotage recovery. Urgency makes your body more physiologically reactive, activating the quick-fire stress response and inhibiting your PFC's ability to think straight.

This is why it can feel so counterintuitive to slow down. So don't be disheartened if when you try to interrupt some of these automatic responses, it feels hard, bordering on impossible. You are fostering bioplasticity which takes repetition and consistency. Each effort counts.

Safety and avoidance behaviours

'Safety behaviour' is a term used in psychology to describe actions that are intended to avert unwanted experiences (e.g. feeling anxious, getting symptoms) but that long term contribute to these experiences. Safety behaviours may be preventative actions like repetitively checking the door is locked to prevent being burgled or avoidance behaviours like not going into work in case you have a flare-up of symptoms. Safety behaviours are generally intuitive responses in situations (or anticipation of situations) that elicit a sense of threat.

Table 2 gives you an impression of what safety and avoidance behaviours look like, but they can be hard to identify. What may be a safety behaviour in one condition may be a necessary behaviour in another situation.[10] For example, taking an extra change of underwear when you have irritable bowel syndrome (IBS) is likely to perpetuate a sense of vulnerability to accidents that generally is not so likely.[11] Therefore, with appropriate assessment, I would move patients with IBS away from this with alternatives to help increase confidence in bowel control. In contrast, for someone with inflammatory bowel disease (IBD) experiencing reduced bowel control because of a flare-up of disease activity, it may be a helpful plan to take spare garments. Working out what is a safety behaviour versus what is necessary behaviour therefore takes

Table 2: Examples of safety and avoidance behaviours seen commonly in physical illnesses, burnout and trauma

Types of safety behaviours	
Behaviour	**Example**
Mental risk minimization	• Lots of time spent calculating what may go wrong • Getting lots of details about plans to create contingency plans
Over-compensating for potential risks	• Bringing extra clothing, equipment or supplies in case of symptoms • Bringing or taking extra medication or supplements in case of symptoms
Checking	• Hyper-focussing on symptoms to monitor for worsening • Paying close attention to bodily processes like stool frequency, smell of urine, sleep timings • Checking for indicators of safety or rescue, e.g. toilets if you're concerned about bowel or bladder symptoms

Micromanaging bodily processes	• Trying to control when you pass a stool or urinate through medication, holding of urges or pre-emptively trying to empty the bladder/bowels • Over-controlling food, diet or fluid intake • Trying to force sleep, monitoring the clock and enforcing strict timings • Inflexible exercise or movement practices

Types of avoidance behaviours	
Avoidance	**Example**
Social withdrawal	• Avoiding places where there will be a lot of people • Avoiding speaking up or drawing attention to yourself • Staying in your own designated safe space
Avoidance of external risk or uncertainty	• Avoiding visiting new areas • Avoiding trying a new hobby or skills • Avoiding trying new treatments
Avoidance of internal risk. (Avoiding doing anything physically, mentally or emotionally that may exacerbate physical symptoms)	• Minimizing physical exertion including acts like shouting or getting emotionally aroused • Avoiding substances that may pose a risk to physical equilibrium. This often involves restrictive diets and aversion to medications • Avoiding thoughts

consideration. This consideration is an important part of the process and it already starts to alter your psychobiology for the better.

How you work out whether to do something or avoid doing something is often automatic and subconscious. Neuroscience research shows that higher order brain regions involved in analytical thinking and cognitive control, referred to as dorsal regions, communicate with the more emotion-centred brain regions, referred to as ventral regions. The dorsal regions help you weigh up pros and cons, whilst the ventral regions help you factor in that intuitive sense of how likely it will be for things to go well (reward anticipation). When there is more uncertainty around the likelihood of things turning out well and there are a lot of factors to consider, your brain becomes more risk averse, relying more on dorsal processes.[12] This physically reduces your brain's ability to factor in the likelihood that things may turn out well. Meanwhile your dorsal regions keep calculating, which is why you can find yourself overthinking.

These processes can keep you stuck in fear-avoidance cycles (Figure 15), where your brain gets less opportunity to experience the rewards gained from action in uncertainty. This builds more fear and more reliance on threat-focussed cognitive processing, increasing fear and keeping avoidance going.

The more threat and anxiety, the more the brain and nervous system can generalize a sense of unsafety to situations where there are no tangible stressors or threats.[13] This is threat mode in action and can have a big impact on your body's regulatory systems.[14] You may feel wired and alert, unable to stop focussing on thoughts that feel pressing.

To try and get relief, so that you can 'switch off', your brain will search for 'safety'. These are cues that it can use to inhibit activity in threat-processing parts of the brain (e.g. amygdala and limbic

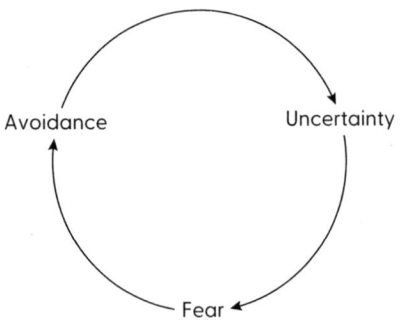

Figure 15: Fear avoidance cycle.

system). Exactly what cues depends on you, the nature of the situation and your prior experiences. If you have post-exertional malaise (extreme exhaustion after movement), you will have had many experiences of feeling gravely depleted after moving your body. Movement becomes a threat and things that amplify that threat will be anything that makes the consequences (fatigue) more likely or more severe. This might be the absence of opportunities to rest, increased temperatures, upcoming activities that will take energy, etc. Your brain will look for cues to reduce concerns about becoming fatigued in the face of movement and if they are sufficient you'll feel less concerned.

What starts as reasonable requests for indicators of safety, can end up snowballing. Knowing that there are places to rest on your planned walk may be enough to alleviate concern beforehand, but your brain ups the demands for reassurance. You go from needing to know that there will be benches, to having to check the exact temperature, checking your heart rate before you leave, getting reassurance from your friend that they are OK if you stop to rest, to planning contingencies for if you do feel symptomatic.

The use of safety behaviours themselves can make symptoms and anxiety about symptoms more likely.[15] This is because the emphasis of the safety behaviour (e.g. checking for benches) to reduce anxiety and prevent fatigue, means that the brain repeatedly associates the absence of these outcomes with the presence of the safety behaviour. It concludes the only reason you didn't get fatigued and feel anxious is because you were able to access benches. Now facing the prospect of going somewhere where you can't know if there will be benches feels more unsafe. Contrast this with the situation where you loosely plan to rest when you need to without the emphasis on benches. You get to the destination; you have a little rest on a side wall or cafe and then you keep going within your capacity. You recognize you are OK. This approach teaches your brain that you can cope in different situations without strict contingencies (i.e. safety behaviours).

Safety behaviours can therefore not only increase anxiety, eroding confidence in your ability to do things without adequate precautions, but also increase the likelihood of symptoms. This has been demonstrated in pain, gut disorders, panic disorder and chronic fatigue syndrome,[16] amongst others. We'll explore the mechanisms of this further in Chapter 5.

Benign emotions

Many societal and cultural messages teach you that negative emotions are toxic experiences to be avoided or battled. These messages shape familial and individual attitudes to emotions, so that you consciously and/or subconsciously believe that 'bad' emotions are bad for you – that they will make you a bad or weak person or will compromise your health. These ideas are myths. Feeling and accepting difficult or 'negative' emotions is healthy – necessary even.[17,18] It is generally the defence mechanisms to emotions that cause issues.

Emotions are natural experiences and arise spontaneously. The beauty of emotions is that they reside in the mind, represented by brain activity patterns *and* they reside in the body reflected by physical sensations, changes in nervous system communication and changes in organ functioning (e.g. heart rate increases, spasms in the colon).[19] Most recent research suggests that you intuitively bunch together these signals, emitted across body systems, into coherent emotional experiences.[20,21] This is a form of multisensory integration. This process is similar to how your brain integrates information to shape your experience of eating. Your brain combines inputs across multiple tastebuds, each with a slightly different role in encoding different elements of taste (e.g. sweet, sour, bitter, salty) in addition to information about the texture, smell and visual appearance of food. In this way, a crispy slice of toast with melting butter elicits multiple senses, potentially strong enough to drive you to act (eat the toast or buy bread to make toast later).

With emotions, in some situations, there will be a loud chorus of senses informing your perception or compelling you to act. If you've ever walked in a dark, unfamiliar and deserted area, you may have felt the pulsing adrenaline and fearful sense that sees you quicken your pace, while your mind races that you need to *'hurry up because you are vulnerable'*. This is an example of a coherent emotional experience communicated across all the modalities to give a clear message to you. In this situation, you may be able to easily identify the emotional experience as 'fear' or 'unease'.

In other situations, elements of the emotional chorus may not feel so clear or coherent. This can cause confusion or disconnection from your experience or even your sense of self. For example, the ongoing experience of pain or physical discomfort can dull your sense of pleasure, meaning that things don't feel as joyful. In the absence of other strong emotional cues like feeling very sad with the tug in your heart or stomach, it can be hard for your brain to paint a clear picture of your emotional state. And yet, you are feeling something that is just below the consciousness that your mind can easily tell you isn't 'quite right' or 'you don't like'.

Making sense of your emotions as a chorus of different mind–body processes helps you to become more familiar with your emotional landscape. From here, you can develop ways of working with your emotions and the biological processes intertwined with them to nurture yourself and your body. Developing the ability to home into different emotional frequencies opens options for responding optimally, ultimately making your body feel safe and nipping in the bud that over-reactivity it can be prone to. We'll explore this more in Chapter 6.

In symptom spirals, feelings may be caused by the situation, physical sensations or an ongoing mood state that has been influenced by various things along the way. As with every other element in the spiral, the precise sequence between emotional experiences and other parts of the spiral doesn't matter so much. It has a two-way relationship with everything else. What is important is how you meet your emotions.

Meeting your emotions means allowing yourself to feel your feelings. Open and compassionate permission to feel, physiologically regulates emotions as reflected in brain imaging studies and measures of autonomic nervous system activity.[22,23]

Unfortunately, difficult emotions like sadness, anger or fear are often met with resistance. Fighting or resisting feelings tends to increase emotional dysregulation and, with that, bodily dysregulation.[24] Resisting feelings also tends to lead to destructive behaviours. These may be unhealthy habits (e.g. drinking, impulsive eating, smoking), disconnecting social behaviours (e.g. angry words, withdrawal) or pressurized over-compensatory behaviours (e.g. over-working, people pleasing). These destructive behaviours perpetuate symptom spirals, entrenching mind–body disharmony.

By far the most common and normalized responses to difficult emotions is emotional suppression, which has been shown to impede immune system function, alter nervous system processes and even change the gut microbiome.[25,26] There are different ways of emotionally suppressing:

- **Blanking out** – Your brain has a nifty defence mechanism of helping you disconnect from your feelings automatically when they are uncomfortable. You reach for your phone, or lose focus. Clients of mine have apologized for 'blanking on the question' when we have got close to something emotionally overwhelming. Over the years, I have become better at recognizing this brain-quirk in action. It offers an exit ramp that my clients aren't even aware they are taking.
- **Pushing down** – Pushing down feelings takes a little more effort and conscious awareness. Often it is done for a greater

sense of good. Ideas like 'I'll upset them' or 'it will make me feel worse' or 'it will harm my health', make it seem like a good idea to deny your feelings. When this happens there is a disconnect between what you are thinking/doing and how you are emotionally and physically feeling. This can create a confusing environment within the body that contributes to threat mode and allostatic load. Physical symptoms that can manifest as a result of this include: increased pain, bowel urgency, bladder issues, fatigue, headaches and recurrent infections.

- **Intellectualizing** – Intellectualizing is one of the reasons inexpertly delivered CBT can be problematic. Intellectualizing involves trying to out-rationalize your feelings so that you persuade yourself not to feel a particular way about something. Of course, that can also be a highly effective form of emotion regulation. If I don't get a job I went for, rather than continuing to feel intensely disappointed, I can realistically tell myself that there will be other opportunities that might even be better suited. I may highlight the downsides of the job I went for to help myself take solace in not getting it. That is all entirely healthy. Intellectualizing is the tendency to use these sorts of strategies repetitively and overbearingly, leaving little to no space for being allowed to *feel* feelings.

At the opposite end of the spectrum to emotional suppression is the experience of feeling inextricably intertwined with your emotions. I will refer to this as 'emotional overidentification'. From this place, everything is perceived through the veil of feelings, which dictate most or all choices. How you feel becomes one of the primary things you attend to and that inform your decisions, over and above other factors. For example, you may feel grumpy and not comfortable in your own skin and then get a request from a friend to meet up. When overly identified with grumpy feelings, it will overshadow lots of other factors that may make you say yes. Things like the benefit of fresh air, connection and new perspective in leaving the house. Instead, you will easily identify that you don't feel good which may make it a foregone conclusion to decline the offer. Your feelings informing your perspective and thoughts are called 'emotional reasoning'.

If you are feeling exposed right now, identifying with many of these ways of dealing with emotions, let me assure you this is a good thing! Just the awareness of how you are processing emotions can help to interrupt automatic neural pathways that keep you (and your body) reactive. The other thing you should know is that we need to rely on these methods of processing emotions sometimes. You are not doing damage by using them. You only have so much capacity for intentional emotion processing. In Chapter 5, you'll be introduced to more emotion processing options for mind–body harmony.

Brain-spamming thoughts

A lot of wellness media demonizes the experience of 'negative thoughts', encouraging you to cleanse your mindset by thinking positively and persuading yourself to disbelieve unpleasant thoughts. This, I'm afraid, is a terribly inaccurate abstraction from CBT. When you are told to repetitively ignore thoughts or cultivate a mindset that sees only solutions, thereby discounting problems, you can end up emotionally suppressing as just described.

Much like with emotions, thinking is potentially quite benign. You have an insurmountable amount of thoughts each day. Although not as many as commonly cited, 50,000–100,000 (which as far as I can see has no scientific origin), it is estimated that you have around 6,200 thoughts a day.[27] These thoughts are the product of your brain churning data and calculations from internal and external experiences to make sense of things. During the process of these calculations, you will have many thoughts that you don't need to consciously pay attention to. I call this 'brain spam'. Many thoughts are neutral (some are nonsense), however the thoughts you become keenly aware of are the scary thoughts. Or thoughts that require actioning. This allows your brain to automatically prioritize without you consciously having to sift through thousands of thoughts. (And you thought sifting through emails was bad!) Simply put, nothing else would get done.

The problem with this, however, is that when your body is depleted, and your various systems (nervous system and regulatory systems) are working to try and find equilibrium, the brain becomes fine-tuned to information that may affect this balancing act. For example, if you have been recovering from burnout after a prolonged period of being overwhelmed with job demands, your brain is going to home in on any indication that you are coming up to, or past, your capacity. That will span contextual cues (the degree of work and how hard tasks are) and sensory information (how tired you feel, how able to concentrate). This means that thoughts related to these potential threats will be given priority in your consciousness. You'll then notice how much time it has taken you to finish a task and the interpretation that you are not concentrating well enough will gather steam. Before you know it, more of your brain space is taken up by these threat-related thoughts, driving emotions like anxiety, overwhelm or resignation.

Common thinking patterns that come from your brain in threat mode are listed in Table 3. These thinking patterns can create or heighten difficult emotions, increase your behavioural reactivity and even elicit physical sensations.

For example, if you are having a flare-up of pain that means you have to cancel plans, you may have an all-or-nothing thought (*I never get to enjoy plans*) fuelling frustration and anxiety. These feelings give rise to more threat-mode thinking patterns like fortune telling (*I'll have to cancel all my plans this weekend*) and mind reading (*My friends all think I'm a weak loser*), intensifying

Table 3: Common thinking patterns that keep mind and body communicating fearfully and reactively		
Threat-mode thinking patterns	**Description**	**Example**
Foretelling the future	Imagining what is likely to happen based on the information present now, with emphasis on the negative and troubling aspects	Getting a pain 3/10 that is new and thinking 'this will get much worse'
Emotional reasoning	A perspective or outlook that is primarily informed by how you are feeling emotionally	Feeling low and unmotivated and thinking 'I won't make plans because I won't feel up to them'
All-or-nothing thinking	Assuming that things fall into a dichotomy of being one way or another	'If I don't get as much enjoyment as I usually do, there is no point'
Mind reading	Believing that you know what someone else is thinking.	Needing to cancel plans and having the thought 'They will be angry'
Self-criticism	Placing blame on yourself and reprimanding yourself for falling short of an assumed standard, action or principle	'If I had tried harder I wouldn't have got into this situation'

emotions. Such thoughts and feelings may make you more likely to ignore messages and stay in bed, in turn making some of the thoughts feel even more believable. As this is happening, your brain has detected the culprit – your pain – and is closely monitoring it. This can elicit more pain. The more pain you feel, the more these thoughts feel factual and the more upsetting the whole experience is.

Thoughts can represent a threat in themselves. They can be threatening because they elicit fear or worry about your well-being or safety (e.g. *my symptoms will get worse* or *people think I'm odd*). They can also be threatening because they contradict your values.

For example, having resentful thoughts about friends being carefree when you are so unwell, can make you feel like you are a bad person. Or having a thought about it being easier if you ceased to exist, might make you alarmed because you wouldn't want to hurt yourself. The mere appearance of these thoughts in your consciousness can activate the threat-processing centres in your brain and cause you extreme distress. Distress may make you focus on the thoughts more, questioning why you thought that or reasoning your way out of it. You may also respond to your thoughts by trying to avoid or suppress them, using all the influence you have with your PFC to banish the thoughts. This takes a lot of energy and research shows that trying to suppress thoughts often makes them more likely to pop up.[28]

'Intrusive thoughts' are thoughts that pop in, unwanted and with high emotional impact. They are common in anxiety disorders like obsessive compulsive disorder (OCD) and health anxiety, but most people have them. Common intrusive thoughts include having thoughts about swerving your car into traffic, pushing people or jumping off the train platform, and leaving your home unlocked. Up to 77% of people surveyed had experienced one or more of these thoughts.[29]

As with emotions, the thought itself is less of an issue than the reaction to it. Remember that your brain is constantly churning through information and coming up with thousands of thoughts per day. That means you cannot be responsible for your automatic thoughts. It also means thoughts can be left to pass and dissipate. Although easier in theory than action, when you start to work with your body to calm biological threat-mode processes, it becomes more accessible. Chapter 4 will help you to do just that.

Situational factors

In symptom spirals, there are two elements: the external situation and the internal response (the spirals). Both have a massive impact on your experience. Whilst it is empowering and important to work on the internal response where you have more control, it is just as important to acknowledge the impact of the situation or environment you are in. If you don't, you can end up elevating expectations of yourself unfairly, causing more stress and self-blame. For example, I've seen people working in very hostile environments, who have been bullied and ostracized, turn in on themselves, assuming that they are the problem and grinding themselves down by working even harder. In Chapter 1, I explained how stress can become normalized and familiar. This can make it hard for you to discern when you are in environments that are actually incredibly hard, if not impossible, to feel safe in: hostile workplaces, abusive relationships, unstable home environments, etc.

Although not always clear cut, the important thing is to be open to exploring how your environment and social setting might be having an impact on your sense of safety. More on this in Chapter 7.

Interrupting your spirals

Perhaps you have already spotted patterns you resonate with. Maybe you are already even coming up with ideas of alternative ways to approach situations. Hopefully, you feel clearer about how your brain is automatically calculating what is happening in your body, how you should respond and how this can create psychobiological loops that keep symptoms going.

In this chapter you have learnt:

- What symptom spirals are and how they can create psychobiological loops that keep symptoms stuck and/or worsening
- What patterns of behaviours and thoughts can drive symptom spirals
- Why it is the defences against emotions rather than the emotions themselves that can keep spirals going long term.

The next chapter is going to introduce you to the first step in moving from threat to safety. Before you do this, you need to map out your own symptom spirals so that you can personalize these strategies to your experience.

Use the exercise below to map out some spirals.

> **Use the symptom spiral framework (page 111) to capture three to five of your own examples from the past and from situations arising across the coming week or two.***
>
> At the end of the week, note the themes of thoughts, emotions, physical experiences and responses. Consider these questions:
>
> - What do you notice?
> - What relationship do you notice between the different parts of your spiral?
> - Did noticing the spirals change your experience of it? How?
> - Do you have any initial thoughts about what small changes you might make to help you meet your goals (Introduction)?

---

* You can download a worksheet at www.healthpsychologist.co.uk/itsallinyourbody

CHAPTER 4

Biology balancing behaviour

Years on from being resigned to my miserable fate in therapy, I was inspired again. At this point, and despite my urologist's foreboding warning that the stress of moving may make symptoms worse, I'd left my job, moved to London and was studying for my master's in health psychology. My symptoms were actually decidedly better. Not gone, but better. But the fact that they weren't gone nagged at me. I'd ricocheted from passive resignation to over-control. I was on 'clean diet' number two, drinking home-blended green smoothies, taking multiple supplements that had the hint of a promise of helping my bladder, and I was militantly exercising. As much as I admire my dedication, with hindsight I was taking on far too much responsibility for my bladder. Although day by day I was highly functional, there were times I'd rage or despair, breaking down in tears as I wondered why things weren't changing when I was trying so hard. I was still fixated on the magic fix. The fact that all my endeavours were falling short of magically fixing things was causing immense stress and bodily reactivity. It was a year or two later, having been immersed in my PhD and research role learning about the transformative effects of pacing and acceptance whilst continuing my mindfulness practices, that I mastered the balance of pacing my efforts to nourish my body while letting go of what I could not control. This allowed my body to go at its own pace and, ultimately, my symptoms to completely subside.

In this chapter, you will be presented with many options for working with your body and the psychobiological processes you have been learning about. This will feel different to other chapters in its practicality, with an array of evidence-based practices and strategies. Some will be more relevant than others for you and your symptoms. Use the symptom spirals you mapped out in the last chapter to inform which approaches are best tailored to your experiences. By the end of this chapter, you'll have a clearer picture of how to work with your body to aid homeostasis. We'll start with the fundamental foundations for the health of your regulatory systems and then bring in ways to enhance interoceptive awareness. From there you'll be guided on small day-to-day tweaks you can implement for reduced bodily reactivity and depletion, and increased sense of safety. Most importantly, remember, there is a balance to be struck between the empowerment of having choices and the pressurizing sense of 'it's all on you'. Taking things gradually, with an experimental approach, can make trying new things feel safe and not overwhelming.

Before you dive in, check in with yourself. How do you feel after the last chapter? What stands out to you so far? You might not be ready to put things into practice but would like to get an idea what doing so might look like. That's OK. Allow yourself permission to take it step by step without knowing how everything will unfold.

Supporting your regulatory systems

As you may recall, you have four core regulatory systems: neuroendocrine, cardiovascular, metabolic and immune system. They are designed to work in harmony to keep your body in balance (homeostasis) and your health intact. The balance is tipped by many things inherent in the experience of illness, chronic stress/burnout or trauma. When you've been trying lots of things to improve your health and feel like you are not where you want to be, your brain can trick you into thinking that nothing you've been doing is worthwhile. It can also make you believe that the basics aren't that important. I've had clients who have tried restrictive diets or sophisticated biometric tracking, later abandoning the *basics* of healthy eating or bodily check-ins along with the diets and biometrics.

From the basics of hydrating, through to the slightly more onerous, such as moving or investing in social connection, some of the simplest things are still the most important. They can get deprioritized by the brain because they are not *the* 'magic fix'. Deprioritization can happen stealthily without you even realizing that you're no longer drinking as much water or eating as regularly and so, when you get a surge of symptoms, you might not readily make the link. For this reason, I thought it important to include 'the basics' for helping regulatory systems to balance things.

Remember, allowing yourself flexibility as you establish habits is fundamental. It prevents mounting pressure that activates threat mode.

- **Diet** – A diet with a rich variety of grains, pulses, spices, fruits, vegetables, along with healthy fats and protein, provides the body with what it needs. This is known as the 'Mediterranean diet' and this is what I recommend as a guide for eating because of the extensive benefits to the gut microbiome, immune system and cardiovascular system.[1,2] How you eat is important too. You might underestimate the importance of regularity in eating and the impact of portion sizes. Keeping eating habits consistent helps the gut get into a routine and looks after your blood sugar levels (and with that the metabolic system).*
- **Hydration** – If your urine is yellowy or brown and smells a lot, you need to hydrate more. The recommended fluid intake

---

* If possible, I recommend seeking tailored guidance from an accredited dietitian with experience of your particular health condition if you have one.

for adults is around 8 cups a day (about 1.5–2 litres). For some, urine is clearish when drinking less than that, in which case you're probably good. However, others may need more than 8 cups, especially if in hot environments or exercising a lot. Keeping hydrated can be difficult. Small things like aversion to gulping or drinking cold drinks when it is cold, can make you naturally avoid hydrating. As with eating, finding a way to make drinking consistent and minimally invasive helps to reach hydration goals. This may be a couple of sips of water from a bottle each hour, preventing bloating and bladder irritation.

- **Movement** – Movement is one of the biggest protectors of regulatory system function and mental health.[3,4] Movement is not necessarily high intensity or even moderate intensity exercise. It includes activities that keep you mobile and flexible, with some variations in heart rate. It is important to prioritize bodily movement according to your own capacity. This can feel particularly distressing and hard to figure out when mobility and fitness is impacted by health issues. We'll explore how to navigate this in a moment.
- **Sleep** – You are probably aware of the importance of sleep. This awareness can also make it harder to access sleep if you worry about not hitting that magic number of hours each night. In Chapter 2, I introduced the concept of sleep homeostasis and in the next section I'll introduce you to how you may utilize this to benefit your sleep.
- **Mental stimulation** – It's common knowledge that keeping your body agile and flexible is good for your health, but the same is true for your mind. Mental stimulation in this context refers to challenging your brain to learn and develop by engaging in cognitively demanding activities (like learning new skills or knowledge). Doing the same things over again, defaulting to previously formed habits and relying on barely consciously formed assumptions can keep you stuck in

symptom spirals, which negatively impacts your health and emotional wellbeing.
- **Strong bonds** – Humans are innately communal beings. Even if you identify as an introvert, strong relationships and sense of connection are integral to your sense of wellbeing and overall health. Relationships may be taken for granted or seen as happenstance. However, your social experiences are something you can influence and invest in. This takes relationship maintenance, difficult conversations, effort and exploration. This doesn't always come easily, but it feeds into your neuroendocrine and immune system in a big way. More on this in Chapter 7.

Additionally, addressing habits that compromise your health is a must. This includes excessive alcohol consumption, binge-eating or highly sugary or fatty diets, drug use or self-harm. These things are not easy to address alone, and I always encourage people dealing with these issues to get support.*

Architecting your sleep

'Sleep architecture' is the scientific term for the natural structure of your sleep which moves through different sleep stages (Table 4).[5] There are four stages of sleep each serving a different purpose for your body, from memory consolidation to cellular regeneration and healing. Understanding the body's natural flexible response to sleep deprivation, and how it utilizes sleep architecture to adjust the quality and structure of your sleep to optimize recovery, can help you to enhance this natural process. This moves away from ideas about owing your body sleep when you have missed out on it (sleep debt), that can make you feel more anxious and pressured to

---

* Signposting for support www.healthpsychologist.co.uk/itsallinyourbody

Table 4: Sleep stages	
Sleep stage	**Function**
Stage 1 – Lightest sleep	To transition from wakefulness to sleep. That 'dozy' state of drifting off
Stage 2 – Light sleep	To stabilize sleep and help memory processing
Stage 3 – Deep sleep	A slow brainwave state that is vital to physically restore the body
Stage 4 – Rapid eye movement (REM) sleep	This is when you experience vivid dreams. This stage of sleep is crucial for memory consolidation and emotion regulation
When you move into each sleep stage depends on you, your natural baseline, your sleeping environment and if your body has missed out on sleep. You move through stages 1 to 4 and then go back round again multiple times during your sleep.	

sleep. Fixation on 'making up for lost sleep' can prevent your brain from switching into sleep mode, because it feels alarmed at the prospect of more potential 'damage' if you don't sleep.

Where it can, the brain *will* increase your total sleep time, but it puts its best foot forward by altering *how* you sleep. Sleep studies show that sleep deprivation results in your brain automatically compensating by increasing the amount of time you are in deep sleep (the stage that is crucial for physical restoration and memory consolidation).[6] Other studies show that you move into REM sleep more easily following periods of sleep deprivation, to help restore cognitive function and mood regulation without needing to catch up on every hour of lost sleep.[7]

The other way your body helps you when you have missed out on sleep, is by making you fall asleep quicker and wake up less.[8] Many of you may be rolling your eyes right now, muttering, 'Sure, wouldn't that be nice!' but here's the important caveat. When left to this process, your body *can* do this for you. This is where symptom spirals get in the way. Concerns about repercussions of sleep deprivation create emotional and physiological stress. In that state of stress and alertness, your brain takes the opportunity to reel off other matters of urgency. This spiral prevents natural sleep architecture.

To help your body do what it is designed to do, here are some principles:

- **Comfort compromise** – Rather than making sleep the intention, make it comfort. Play a game with your brain to feel as comfortable and snug as possible. Any time your brain turns itself to the question of sleep, come back to all the things that make you feel comfortable and comforted.
- **Sleep aids** – Give the brain cues for comfort to let it know it doesn't have to be alert. This might be having a bedtime drink like camomile, scents like lavender, diffusers with warm glowy lights and big fluffed-up pillows. If, in the beginning, your brain is too busy, you might find it useful to use some background noise to pacify that need to be processing something while not feeling too stimulated. 'Pink noise' is a type of sound that contains all frequencies that humans can hear, but with a balanced energy distribution giving it a softer, deeper and more natural quality compared to white noise. Pink noise can reduce brainwave activity, slowing down that fast mind and enhancing deep sleep.[9] Sounds of rainfall, wind, ocean waves, steady heartbeat, the gentle rustling of leaves, are all types of pink noise.
- **Avoid or minimize naps*** – Napping, especially too close to your bedtime, disrupts your body's internal clock (circadian rhythm) and it prevents a build-up of adenosine

---

* If your body is depleted and you have increased sleep needs, you may require naps. It is important to assimilate this guidance with your own bodily intuition and medical advice. We will explore bodily intuition further in this chapter.

(a neurotransmitter that increases during the day to create sleep pressure – your need to sleep). This can make it harder for you to drop off to sleep later. The more you resist napping, the easier the task is for your brain to get you off to sleep at bedtime when you've been losing out.

- **Morning routine; less is more** – Your morning routine is just as important as your evening routine. Hitting the snooze button can create erratic sleep–wake times, making it harder for your body to get into a rhythm. Try to maintain a regular hour window of waking each day (e.g. 8–9 a.m.). Don't confuse feeling groggy and tired with the need to sleep in. Feeling groggy is often because you have woken up from a deeper sleep because your body has optimized your sleep, thereby reducing the amount of light sleep. If you can get moving into your morning routine, your brain gets into a faster brainwave state and this grogginess can recede. Having a rewarding morning routine can help get you started with this. Create breadcrumbs that coax you into the day. Things like setting the coffee machine to come on so that you wake up to the smell of coffee, or having a hot soapy bath planned or a quick jaunt with your dog.
- **Tailor your sleep times to your natural body clock** – Advances in research have debunked the idea we all need a magic eight hours and run on the same clock.[10] Some people are natural night owls, whilst others are early risers. And, rather than one long shift, there are also people who naturally sleep in two phases (biphasic) as seen in cultures that have siestas. You might already have an idea of your natural body clock, in which case explore your options for working with it to whatever degree you can. If you're not sure, then note when you naturally start to feel tired (whether or not you sleep) and when you naturally wake up without intervention. You can use this to guide the sleep and wake times you set for yourself.

Recognizing where your body is at

Recognizing where your body is at involves fine-tuning interoceptive awareness (page 61). Building interoceptive awareness improves mental health and physical symptoms in chronic conditions like multiple sclerosis, stroke recovery, diabetes and chronic pain. A programme that involved experientially building interoceptive awareness for people with MS, led to improved balance and coordination.[11,12] In stroke rehabilitation, bodily awareness training improved the recovery of motor functions[13]. In diabetes, interoceptive awareness has been shown to improve blood glucose control, through tailored interoceptive blood glucose perception training.[14] For individuals with chronic pain, a mix of mind–body therapies have been shown to enhance interoceptive awareness and reduce pain intensity and pain-related disability.[15] Inherent to all these interventions was a fine-tuning of the awareness of bodily signals while remaining regulated.

You are going to build a foundation for fine-tuning this awareness now, starting by building interoceptive awareness specifically of your ANS, which is involved in the quick-fire stress response (page 41). I have emphasized that activation of the ANS is healthy. You may recall that there are sub-branches of the ANS, the SNS and the PNS. The two work together to help you activate to meet demands (including stress) and come back to an equilibrium when it is safe to be at rest. At least theoretically.

A healthy ANS sees a lot of SNS activity daily to differing degrees. The important thing is that your PNS can counterbalance where necessary. The experience of ongoing stress, physical symptoms and mood disorders can mean the ANS gets stuck in one 'nervous system state' or another and seldom reaches balance. In the nervous system barometer (Figure 16), three states are depicted:

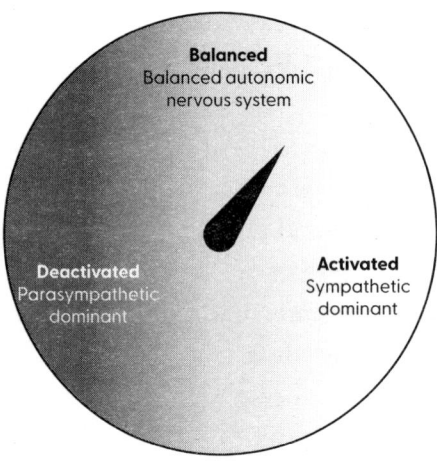

Figure 16: The nervous system barometer, illustrating the spectrum between the three nervous systems states that you can transition across.

- **Activated** – At most activated, your SNS is actioning the quick-fire stress response. Stress hormones are circulating, your blood is pumping, heart racing and your organs and muscles are responding to the hormones.
- **Deactivated** – At most deactivated, there is an extreme form of parasympathetic dominance depressing metabolic and cognitive functions, physically impeding your ability to engage in activity. This often happens when your body is exhausted and can't sustain the sympathetic response or is under extreme stress.
- **Balanced** – When at rest, with the PNS and SNS at balance, you have capacity to activate if needed but you can disengage from demands. This state is not always pleasant, it can be neutral and even a little boring. As long as that boredom isn't experienced intensely negatively in a symptom spiral full of frustrated thoughts, it is still restorative.

Each of these states blend into each other in a spectrum* and

---

* Colour version available at www.healthpsychologist.co.uk/itsallinyourbody

often you will find yourself somewhere between two of the states, which is entirely healthy. This is part of fine-tuning interoceptive awareness. Between balanced and activated, you may start to observe the more subtle physical experiences of activation in different situations. For example, the fluttery, bubbly feeling of excitement when you are looking forward to something or the mild-fizzing, head-blocky feel of building pressure as you tackle your to-do list. Noticing these subtle experiences of activation can help your body feel safer when there are interoceptive signals of activation, like increased heart rate that may otherwise cause spikes in anxiety or agitation.

Exploring the subtle signs of mounting fatigue/exertion between activated and deactivated states can cue you to give yourself a break. Giving yourself a break can potentially move you from heading towards deep deactivation where you feel numb, heavy and exhausted, to falling somewhere healthily between balance and activated again (Figure 17). A healthy ANS is one full of fluctuations across the barometer.

Across the nervous system states, you can have many different

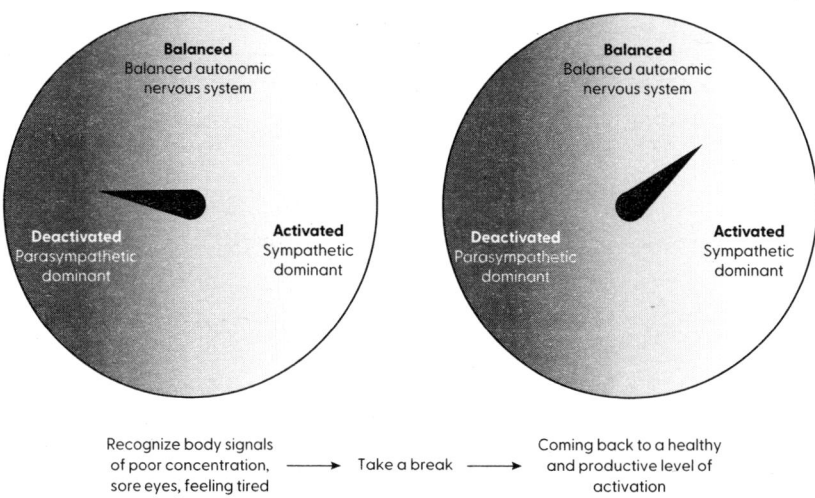

Figure 17: An example of change in nervous system state by recognition of bodily signals in one state allowing appropriate action (taking a break).

physical and emotional experiences. Being in the heart of the activated state when you are at a job interview, with the feeling it is going badly, can look very different to being in the same state when you are being told something upsetting by a doctor. Table 5 gives some examples of physical and emotional feelings across the different states. This is neither a definitive nor exhaustive list. Every person varies.

The practice detailed next aims to help you build and fine-tune your awareness of subtle bodily signals (interoceptive awareness),

Table 5: Nervous system states		
Nervous system states	**Physical feelings**	**Emotions**
Activated	Heart racing Shallow breaths Tight chest Agitation Racing thoughts hard to pin down Urgency Tension Darting attention	Stressed Frustrated Angry Scared Anxious Motivated Determined Excited
Shut down (deactivated)	Heaviness/immobilized Slow brain Brain fog Aches and pains Tension Fatigue Feeling unwell Shaky/weak	Sad Helpless Out of control Despair Dread Uninspired Apathy Numb
Balanced	Satisfactorily tired Energized Loose Light In sync with healthy body cues (hunger/thirst) Relaxed	Content Safe Happy Joy Satisfied Interested Engaged

so that you are better able to hear your body when it whispers, thereby preventing it from needing to shout in the future. Like much else in this book, this is not a quick hack, but a habitual practice that has the power to harness bioplasticity and change your relationship with your body to one of trust.

As you do the practice, your brain may skip ahead: *I'm hearing what it's saying, but what should I do now that I hear it?* Rest assured that you are doing plenty to support your body simply by listening. This very process can enhance your regulatory system's ability to balance allostatic load and reduce threat-mode activation. Rather than jumping ahead to making big changes, slowly integrate these in as you become more familiar with the content of this chapter and those that follow. You may like to use page 100 to draft up ideas for stepping-stone goals as you go.

Suggested practice: recognizing nervous system states

Over the course of one to two weeks, spot different nervous system states and make a log of when you find yourself in them. You can use the template below to do so. In each column make note of your answers to these questions:

- What does it physically feel like in your body?
- How does it feel emotionally?
- Do you notice any urges, impulses or actions?

Situation	Approaching or in activated state	Approaching or in deactivated state	Approaching or in balanced state

Getting the balance of activity right

We've considered how your body can be predisposed to lurch between pushing you hard, at risk of overdoing things, or backing off and withdrawing too much. These lurches contribute to dysregulation and allostatic load. That's why it is so important for all healing goals to navigate towards balance. Balance doesn't mean always being zen and having meticulously planned routines. Pacing is a common evidence-based approach to balancing energy for persistent fatigue.[16] It involves monitoring how much you have physically exerted yourself and ensuring counterbalances. In clinical practice, I've found that pacing regimens promoting focus on strict measures of physical exertion (e.g. thirty minutes of walking 'no more, no less') can disrupt healthy interoceptive awareness, creating fearful hypervigilance. This can make you take overcautious measures to pre-emptively compensate for over-exertion, like lying down for long periods or avoiding socializing or things that may cause stress.

This is why I adapted traditional pacing processes to incorporate recognition of the nervous system states (interoceptive awareness). This process allows you to build more bodily trust, enhance multisensory integration and incorporate flexibility into the stability of routines. It allows the multidimensionality of a given activity, so that you don't see experiences as a dichotomy of depleting or replenishing. For example, seeing a friend can demand some physical and attentional resources, which could cause you to label that activity as 'depleting'. However, the experience of connecting, feeling affection and enjoying leisure time is psychobiologically replenishing. Recognizing the multidimensionality is important to help your body feel safer and stop automatic threat mode that can feed symptom spirals. This better enables you to reach balance.

Using the nervous system pacing diary

Figure 18 is an example of a partially completed nervous system pacing diary that you can download.* It is designed for you to fill in some brief detail each day of what you are doing and your corresponding nervous system states. This will help you further develop interoceptive awareness skills and bodily intuition needed to help your body regulate. It can be particularly illustrative to use colour coding to depict the nervous system states so you can clearly see what states you are most frequently in.

Use the guidance below to help you.

- Each day, pick three to four points in the day to record in brief detail what you have been doing in each hourly box. If you leave it longer than three to four hours, you tend to forget how you were feeling. These intervals create opportunities for you to build the habit and skill of interoceptive awareness.
- Colour code the nervous system states. You can access the coloured barometer online. It shows a spectrum from red (activated), to blue (deactivated), to green (balanced). Colour in shades according to what you have been feeling. The spectrum is important here. For example, you may not have been deep in activated mode as depicted by a red, but approaching activation, depicted by orange or yellow. Using colours can help your brain recognize that sympathetic activation isn't automatically bad or dangerous. This differentiation helps interrupt automatic threat mode activation.
- Make note of 'mini-interrupters'. These are the little micro tasks, activities or experiences that may elicit a state change to replenish you, like moving rooms, having a drink, stopping

---

* Resources at www.healthpsychologist.co.uk/itsallinyourbody

	Monday	Tuesday	Wednesday	Thursday	Friday	Saturday	Sunday
Stress rating	8/10	6/10	4/10	4/10	2/10	3/10	5/10
Symptom rating	7/10	3/10	3/10	3/10	3/10	2/10	4/10
6am – 7am	Wake up routine	Wake up routine	Wake up routine	Wake up routine & Meditate	Wake up routine & Meditate	Sleep	Sleep
7am – 8am	Breakfast	Commute	Breakfast	Breakfast	Argument & work	Sleep	Sleep
8am – 9am	Emails	Admin	Working	Admin	Meeting	Sleep	Sleep
9am – 10am	Working	Working	Working	Admin/Procrastinate	Walk	Breakfast & TV	Breakfast & TV

Figure 18: Example of a partially filled out nervous system pacing diary. The greying reflects where colours have been used to represent the different nervous system states.

a work task to have a chat. You don't need to catch and detail all of them, but it is useful to start detecting them because they can be powerful, as you will see later.
- Each day at a similar time, rate how affected you have been by your symptoms, from 0 (not at all) to 10 (completely). You could have a score per symptom (e.g. fatigue, pain) or you could combine and have one score to depict how affected you've been by symptoms overall. Make it as simple as possible with as few different data points as possible.
- Each day, rate overall distress/mood from 0 (no distress or negative mood state) to 10 (highest distress/negative mood state). It works best to keep it as a general indication of emotional intensity rather than specify feelings at this stage.

Just by consciously paying attention to your experience and interoceptive experiences, you have changed how mind and body are communicating, building trust and reducing reactivity.

Your nervous system profile

After a week or fortnight of recording in your diary, use the reflective prompts in Table 6 to explore areas you may focus on to get more bodily balance. You may find that you fit into one of the following profiles or fall somewhere between them.

The head-firster

Head-firsters run head first into their life and busyness. Often, they're ruled by their 'head' and less so by their body. The to-do list keeps generating and they keep jumping to the demands of it, often successfully and with a sense of achievement but with less awareness of the impact on the body.

A diary of a head-firster will typically feature lots of orange and red shades, illustrative of varying degrees of nervous system

Table 6: Prompts for altering activity for bodily balance

	✓/✗		✓/✗		✓/✗
Are there big blocks of colour indicating large periods of time in one nervous system mode or another?		Do these tend to be big blocks of either activation or deactivation?		Did you forget to seek out balancing activities or experiences?	If two or more ✓ consider what made it hard to experience the balance state more?
Did you have moments of mini-interrupters breaking up nervous system states – even just for a few minutes?		Did you notice an impact on your nervous system state of little breaks or task changes, even if fleeting?		Did you consider filling the diary out to be a mini-interrupter?	If two or more ✗ explore what prevented you from seeking or deriving benefit from mini-interrupters. The symptom spiral framework (page 111) may be helpful to explore this.

Was there clear regularity or routine across your days or week, e.g. sleep–wake times, eating?	✓/✗	Was your sleep specifically regular?	✓/✗	Were your meal times generally regular?	✓/✗	If two or more ✗ explore what made regularity challenging. You might like to generate ideas of what could help establish routine.
Did you notice a relationship between your symptom scores and nervous system states?	✓/✗	Did symptoms have an impact on your nervous system states?	✓/✗	Did your nervous system states have an impact on your symptoms?	✓/✗	If two or more ✓ consider what the nature of the relationship is between these states, your symptom experience and your activity. Chapters 2–4 may help.
Did you notice a relationship between your distress/mood score and nervous system state?	✓/✗	Did your mood have an impact on your nervous system states and/or activity?	✓/✗	Did your nervous system states have an impact on your mood and/or activity?	✓/✗	If two or more ✓ explore how your emotional state, nervous system state and activity are impacting on each other. Use the symptom spiral framework to unpick this (page 111).

activation. Each day will be peppered with lots of tasks and commitments, often running into each other without much of a break. Even recreational activities, designed to restore and replenish, require elevated physical and/or mental exertion. A lot of head-firsters have 'up-tempo' stress relievers, like exercise or socializing, that don't involve too much slowing down or being.

While some head-firsters pride themselves on their structure and schedules, which they can run with military precision, others are more haphazard, finding corners of time to squeeze things into. A lot of my ADHD clients are head-firsters.

Symptom activity and patterns will depend to some degree on what health conditions and symptoms the head-firster has. Generally, there can be a tendency for fluctuating symptoms which can seem completely random, or symptoms that remain average or high across a week. A common experience head-firsters have is that when they do slow down a little, they feel *more* symptoms. Because they have been operating in a predominantly activated mode powered by cortisol and adrenaline, which are pain-suppressors and energy stimulators, when they slow down the PNS activates to restore. This washes out the stress hormones which can get rid of the pain-suppressing effect, meaning that pain flares. It also means that the energy injection has gone and the body tries to restore itself, likely in a depleted state, creating fatigue or lethargy. For those with bowel issues, the activation of the PNS restores digestive processes, which may have been paused or altered during all the activity, and this can kick off cramps, bloating or repeated visits to the toilet.

The observer

In contrast, a diary of an observer may have a much sparser landscape, favouring repetitive activity choices and space in between activating activities. Clients of mine that fit into this profile have often felt embarrassed when completing diaries, apologetically telling me, 'There won't be much in there'. Like the head-firster, the observer spends much time in their head, observing symptoms, analysing experiences, gathering information and trying their best to make the '*right*' decisions. This can mean that they are cautious about doing new things or doing too much. They may have previously been a head-firster and then found themselves impacted by debilitating symptoms that they now wish to avoid at all costs.

Depending on the context and situation of the observer – such as whether they are in work, have social support and how actively they are engaging with healthcare – the dispersion of nervous system states will vary. When there are less urgent demands like appointments or stressful chores, there may be a lot of baseline deactivation (reflected in purply blue hues if you are using the coloured diary). These experiences of deactivation are characterized by feeling numbed, low, lacking pleasure or motivation. For an observer, activities entered in the diary to give a sense of pleasure, like socializing or mooching in shops, may be experienced as activating rather than balancing (depicted by shades of orange or pink rather than yellow or green if you are using the colour-coded diary). This is because the activation required to do them automatically feels mildly threatening to the brain and body, changing the physical experience of the activity.

Regularity of the basics like bedtime, waking and eating can vary across observers, with a tendency to have more time in bed or sleeping on weekends. Usually this is related to a sense of needing to replenish the body by catching up on rest. Symptom patterns again will vary depending on the health condition, but often, conversely to head-firsters, symptoms increase in relation to increased activation. This can in part be explained by the autonomic activation that can heighten the activity of networks that are primed to detect threat, causing upregulation in nerve signalling, increased heart rate and circulation of stress hormones, resulting in changes to organ and muscle functioning that can exacerbate symptoms.

The boom/buster

The boom/buster is someone who oscillates between over-exertion and withdrawal/depletion. A boom/buster will have a diary full of colourful blocks, going from one extreme of activation (red or bright orange), closely followed by deactivation (blues and purples). The boom/buster may have more access to periods of balance (green or yellow hues) than the other two profiles, but again experiences these moments in blocks rather than sprinklings throughout the week.

With the oscillating activity patterns, symptoms also tend to vary. A boom/buster may experience the same phenomenon head-firsters have, of an increase in symptoms when resting or depleted, leading to increased withdrawal in an effort to recover. Withdrawal can increase internal pressure, so when they do start to feel better, they throw themselves back into activity much like a head-firster. A lot of my clients with IBS are boom/busters and experience fluctuating bowel symptoms to match.

Tweaking your activity to get more balance

Regular sleep/wake and eating windows

Use the guidance on page 135 to prioritize increasing regularity across the following: sleep, eating, hydration, movement, social connection. Prioritize in that order according to where you lack regularity. For instance, if you have regular sleep but are not eating, prioritize that. If you have both, focus on hydration. To begin with, pick just one area to focus on.

Reducing doing and increasing being

Society encourages you to be in a state of doing as often as possible. That means being active, achieving, ticking things off. 'Being' can be deprioritized as a luxury to be had *only* if you've done everything you need to do. This reduces your opportunity to rebalance. Small pauses, slow mornings, time spent daydreaming is eroded in favour of squeezing things in. Research shows that allowing yourself to 'be', without emphasis on achieving or figuring things out, activates a network of brain areas called your default mode network (DMN). Opportunity for DMN activation facilitates restoration of bodily balance through nervous system regulation, emotion processing and physiological recovery.[17]

If you recognize a scarcity of 'being' moments, start small. Each day, intentionally cultivate small moments (minutes even) to just be without any extra stimulation. Daydream, mind wander, look out of the window, sit with a drink or whatever you fancy. As you do, you are physically helping your body to establish more balance – as inconsequential as it may seem. Small moments stack up. You can use these moments of being as 'mini-interrupters' to break up big durations of being in a particular nervous system state. Swap phone use for small moments of being.

Feeding your body positive experiences

The societal emphasis on achievement and doing means that pleasure or experiences just for the sake of feeling good feelings (interest, pleasure, playfulness) get deprioritized. Many of my clients tell me how hard they find it to intentionally engage in just three pleasurable or replenishing experiences each day. My suggested antidote is simple in theory and tends to be harder in practice. Prioritize, even pre-plan, activities each day that are centred around nourishment, pleasure or catharsis in some way that can act as 'mini-interrupters' to recalibrate nervous system states (Table 7). You're not aiming for 10/10 pleasure or sense of nourishment. Even a 1/10 counts. Just like allostatic load, these moments of counterbalance stack up, making your body more able to reach homeostasis.

Don't underestimate the importance of this. By doing it consistently, you are training your brain to attend to positive experiences which help to recalibrate threat-detecting and negativity biases.[18,19] This is an important element of helping you and your body feel safe. If you find it is hard to experience positive feelings in relation to doing pleasant things, don't worry. Research shows that doing it anyway starts to change how your brain is experiencing these things, increasing your access to positive feelings.[20,21] In Chapter 5, I'll introduce you to the concept of savouring which can help with this.

Increasing doing

If you recognize it is important to do more of certain activities, this doesn't necessarily mean you have to squeeze more in. Consider where you can swap things out rather than just add more to your to-do list. For example, you may experiment with closing your laptop before 8 p.m. to *make space* for an evening stroll instead of closing your laptop at 8 p.m. and *squeezing in* an evening stroll.

For some, especially those of you feeling vulnerable and unsure of your physical or emotional capacity, the prospect of doing more can feel scary. My suggestion is to first focus on regularity and establishing a baseline of activities that feel safe for you using the previous practices. From here, if you are noticing high levels of deactivation and a lack of activity, you can then gradually experiment with adding more in. This might be physical activity like walking or stretching. It might be socially focussed, like more time with friends. Or it might be an activity that involves mental exertion like reading or increasing office work hours.

Table 7: Examples of 'mini-interrupters' for nervous system state changes

Activity	Elements to consider when using activities to activate or deactivate to get you closer to balance
Stretches or yoga Small chores Walking Enjoyable hobby done mindfully (e.g. crafts, painting, doodling, writing) Journaling Socially connecting to a level that feels feasible Planning Watering your plants Reading Pet care Breathing Slow-paced yoga Quiet time with minimal stimulation Dumping thoughts on a page Walking Reading Getting lost in fiction or entertainment Getting a drink Eating mindfully (with no extra activity) Looking out of the window Lighting a candle or scent	Duration, intensity, cognitive load, accessibility, feasibility, emotional needs

Start small and avoid extremes. Generally, I suggest that people experiment with gradually increasing frequency and variation of similar activity types, before aiming for increases in duration. For example, adding the option of doing gentle yoga for ten minutes instead of your ten-minute walk would be preferable to trying to increase your walk to thirty minutes at a quicker pace. Sharply increasing the duration of an activity is more likely to lend itself to extreme fluctuations. What we're aiming for is gentle assimilation.

Wherever you start to increase activity of any kind, observe the impact using the nervous system pacing diary. You can compare new diaries with previous ones. Pay attention to how increases of activity are impacting on your mood, nervous system states and symptoms. Give yourself time to assess this (at least a couple of weeks).

Explore whether these changes are reflective of your body's increasing ability to come back to a balance. Don't be deterred if changes aren't linear. In establishing balance, it can be useful to think of it like stepping into a rowing boat on the water. As you step in, everything veers choppily to one side. You have to redistribute your weight a few times before you find that stability and the rocking stops.

Safeness increasing behaviours

I introduced you to the concept of 'safety behaviours' earlier: the things you do to minimize the ever-expanding sense of threat your brain determines there is when threat mode is activated. Although providing short-term relief (perhaps), safety behaviours make your world smaller, further eroding a sense of safety, meaning and enjoyment.

A few months into illness, I had lost my sense of competence. Seeing people socially felt like a huge effort and the toll on my mind and body didn't seem worth it. Even leaving the house felt unsafe, so instead I'd wear the same loose trousers and assortment of jumpers, feeling unclean and stagnant, even when washed. My comfort zone was not comfortable, but it felt safer than the alternative. But this 'comfort' zone created symptom spirals that made me more symptom-focussed, lonely, anxious and ultimately feeling terrible about myself.

When my boyfriend at the time (now husband) patiently coaxed me out of the house to have lunch at a cafe or get a drink in a cosy pub, it wasn't smooth sailing. One of the first times, I ended up running to the toilet horrified by burning pain in my bladder that struck just as our food arrived, and then demanding through tears, that we leave. Another time, we went to a pub, and I stared off into the distance dissociatively musing about how simple the lives of others around us seemed to be. And yet, these experiences and the others that followed laid important groundwork. They made outside the house feel more accessible, even if it wasn't desirable right then. And on some level, there was *some* relief and reward that penetrated my threatened consciousness. I know so, because I still remember the appetizing food that was served although I could not eat it. And the brisk air and blue sky of the day we went to the pub. These experiences were changing how my brain was processing things, even though it didn't feel like it at the time. As mentioned earlier, having these experiences physiologically retrains your brain to be more able to experience positive feelings and reduce threat biases that colour how you see things.[22,23]

Coaxing yourself out of your comfort zone can be difficult to do at first. Approaching it experimentally and addressing the threats your brain is perceiving explicitly can help. You can do this using something called 'behavioural experiments'. These are processes used in CBT to help patients get curious about making changes that feel scary. Experimenting helps recalibrate the brain from high threat level to something more realistic and reassuring.

I will illustrate with a clinical case study:

Freya was bed-bound with fatigue for several months. She could and would get out of bed, but she seldom left her bedroom. She equated sleeping and lying down with safety because she could guarantee that she wasn't asking too much of her body and that would prevent extreme exhaustion. However, she still had very high levels of fatigue when staying in this zone of safety.

We looked at whether she could increase her time out of bed by ten minutes. During that time, she could remain in her bedroom and be sitting down, but she must be out of her bed and not lying down. We agreed if she felt like it, she could try to be in the living room with her family on some of those occasions. She was open to it, but worried that she would get a big spike in exhaustion right after and that this exhaustion would last for days. She also worried this would knock her mood and she would feel depressed and hopeless.

These concerns were predictions we quantified a little more. The anxious brain is generally vague and ambiguous, offering up endless what-ifs. Pinning down the what-ifs helps to recalibrate threat. We quantified the predictions as depicted in Table 8, specifying the perceived likelihood of them.

We then considered whether the experiment felt safe enough or if we should modify it given how high her prediction was for the exhaustion spike and how some days she didn't leave bed at all. We agreed instead that every two days she would leave bed for ten minutes, but this could be broken up into two sets of five minutes.

When I saw her later, she had managed to experiment three times. Although not every two days, this was significant! We then looked at the ratings she'd made and I checked with her whether they had been accurate. The new percentages reflected just how much her brain had overestimated the threat. Although her exhaustion had increased a little on one or two days, it was not to the 10/10 intensity she had predicted. She was also relieved that it hadn't persisted longer than a day and, far from feeling more depressed, she felt more hopeful.

Table 8: Example behavioural experiment sheet

If I am out of my bed for an extra ten minutes each day and spend some of that time in the living room, it will result in the following

Predictions	Predicted likelihood 0% (no chance) to 100% (certain)	Accuracy of prediction 0% (not at all accurate) to 100% (happened exactly as predicted)
A spike of exhaustion moving from baseline exhaustion level (6/10 intensity) to 10/10 intensity	60%	20%
The spike of exhaustion lasting at least three days	50%	10%
Feeling more depressed and hopeless	50%	0%

Creating behavioural experiments

You can use the same processes to help you experiment with getting out of your safety zone. Here's how:

1. What do you want to change and what fears are preventing you from making that change?
2. How can you feasibly, safely and minimally experiment with doing more or less? Consider durations, manner, context and support. Consider starting with short durations or enlisting support (e.g. from partner or friend) to begin with.
3. Once you have identified what your experiment is, clarify what your threat-detecting brain predicts. List the predictions and rate them in terms of likelihood percentages.

4. Do the experiment a few times, reflect back and log outcomes so your brain has a chance to see where there are inaccuracies.
5. Decide what this means for you and what you'd like to do now you have this information. What is more feasible now – even if just a bit?

Hacking your attentional habits

Your focus of attention is the invisible behaviour that no one can see. Your brain in threat-detecting mode affects your attention, increasing hypervigilance that can increase physical symptoms and anxiety. Hypervigilant attention contributes to overall body dysregulation.

You're generally not explicitly taught how to harness or work with your attentional focus and it can feel like it has a will of its own. Where your attention automatically goes and how able you are to focus or harness your attention is impacted by your biology, psychology and social experiences. People with ADHD or autism may experience more amygdala hijacks (page 49) and have more difficulties harnessing the PFC (the key brain region that directs your attention). However neuroplasticity and bioplasticity mean that you can still harness your attention with practice.[24,25]

One particular study examined whether patients who had brain injuries from trauma, stroke, surgery or chemotherapy could recover from attentional deficits and difficulties sustaining and directing attention.[26] Participants received goal-directed attention training which combined mindfulness and goal management techniques (similar to what we have explored in the Introduction). In just five weeks participants showed significant improvements in their ability to focus attention, ignore distractions and sustain their attention on goal-relevant information, thereby enhancing learning and memory. Brain imaging techniques showed neural changes in the attentional processing regions of the brain (including the PFC) reflective of these changes. The striking thing about this study and others like it is that it demonstrates the adaptability of the brain, even in injury.

Increasing attentional influence and working with it could be a book in itself. For now, I've included some foundational practices that help you metaphorically build your brain muscles that enable you to direct your attention. These practices are based on evidenced-neuroscientific processes and psychological interventions.[27]

Attentional issues to target

- **Worry and rumination** – Your attention is repeatedly pulled towards future worries or negative thoughts you have limited/no control over
- **Fearful fixation (hypervigilance)** – Your attention keeps being directed towards salient threats like physical symptoms or specific worry themes (e.g. being let down or judged)
- **Self-focus** – Your awareness of your self – how you are coming across, what you look or sound like – is amplified, thereby increasing self-consciousness.

Playing with your attentional spotlight

Imagine a spotlight in your brain that can point internally or externally. When it points internally it highlights every sense you feel, every evaluative thought you are having about yourself and emotional discomfort. When pointing externally, you can engage with your surroundings more presently. The intensity and harsh light being shed on those internal processes is duller, making them less concerning. Studies show that you can effectively train your spotlight to dial down the shine of the spotlight beam internally.[28,29] When you do, it reduces anxiety, enhances enjoyment and regulates your body's stress response.

We'll come back to working with attention, but at this stage, it is helpful to master a starter practice to help you intentionally influence your attentional spotlight.

The practice:

- Pick a spot where you feel safe, comfortable and relatively confident you won't be disturbed. Take some slow deep breaths to ground yourself.
- Imagine a ruler that runs from all the way deep inside your head and body, internally, to a metre or so in front of you, externally. The furthest external point of this ruler is +3. The most internal part of this ruler (inside your head) is −3. The ruler marks 0 just at your nose where your attentional spotlight is on you and your external surroundings.
- Focus your attention as fully as you can internally (−3) and stay there, noticing what you feel physically, emotionally and any thoughts you are having. Notice if you have a sense of self-consciousness or judgement as you do this. Rate where you manage to plant your attentional spotlight on that ruler (e.g. did you get all the way to −3 or was it more like a −2 or −1?).
- Now move your attention as externally as you can, allowing any thoughts or feelings about yourself to fade into the background. Don't block them out, instead move your attention to whatever grabs you in your surroundings. The light, the temperature, the colours and textures. Perhaps the sounds and general sense of being in the space you are in. Rate where you manage to plant your attentional spotlight on the ruler now.
- Jot down how it felt to be focussed internally versus externally and repeat the exercise.

You can repeat this multiple times in a day or across a week. Each time you do, you are building your brain's ability to move away from threatening thoughts and internal senses. This is helpful for unpleasant symptoms as well as overthinking and social anxiety.

Build this skill by trying it in a slightly more challenging setting (like being outside or at work). You can use this same approach when you are socializing. In these situations, the external focus of attention is on the person, what they are saying and your interaction, rather than your judgement of yourself and awareness of how you are coming across.

Don't do it all

You've learnt a lot of different things in this chapter:

- The basic habits necessary to support your regulatory systems to help the body rebalance, including sleep architecture, regular and nutritionally varied meals, hydration, maintaining low impact movement, mental stimulation and social bonds
- How to recognize physiological nervous system states to guide what you do next
- The principles of nervous system guided pacing
- How to increase a sense of safeness, reducing threat-mode defaults by experimenting with your comfort zone and training your attention.

Don't try to incorporate everything from this chapter at once. It will reduce your ability to stay consistent and get momentum. The 'intention-behaviour gap' is the common phenomenon that setting an intention isn't sufficient for behavioural change. It is not a personal failing; it is another quirk of being a human. Here are some things you can do to close the intention-behaviour gap whilst working out what you want to put into practice from this chapter:

- Pick a specific action to focus on and make it tangible (e.g. I will print out the nervous system diary and log activities for a week)
- Specify why you are doing this and how this is related to your goals (revisit page 27 goals)
- Plan when, how and in relation to what you will be doing the thing you want to do (e.g. every evening at 6 p.m. just before dinner at the kitchen table)
- Mentally rehearse imagery of you doing the thing
- Imagine how you will feel after having done it and how it relates to your goals.

The sense of personal responsibility to heal can be so great it becomes disempowering as you second-guess every decision or rush to try everything. I seemed to stumble into one thing after the other, be it medical approaches like getting my bladder pumped with soothing gel or taking long-term antibiotics, or alternative practices like drinking apple cider vinegar (there were many 'holistic' hypes I tried). I say 'stumbled' because I, like many of the clients who come to see me, had no integrated support in the healthcare system. I was the amateur project manager of my own health, trying to make sense of things and ultimately jumping at the opportunity to find a magic fix. When I became more patient and consistent with my body, my relationship with it improved. Remember it is just as much about what you don't do as what you do. This is fundamental for helping access more balance and regulation in your body.

CHAPTER 5

Feeling yourself better

In that first year of moving to London to study the master's in health psychology, my symptoms much less severe, I was tentatively re-emerging into the world. Before getting ill, socializing was second nature to me. I was the person who rallied up a hundred-plus psychology students on a road trip to Amsterdam. But things were different now. I felt vulnerable and exposed to a hostile world.

One night, I was making an effort to make friends in London. Before, I'd beeline to the bar, grab a drink and throw myself into conversation. But this night, I was weighed down with considerations. I feared the alcohol would make my bladder worse, so every sip felt like I was assaulting my body, and I braced for a sting, with only fleeting relief when it didn't come. My conversation felt off-kilter, disconnected and *boring*. I felt sorry for the people talking to me and redoubled my efforts to make my presence enjoyable, but to no avail.

As my partner and I were walking home on the suburban lamp-lit streets of south London, he casually commented on how friendly the women had been. Out of nowhere, I felt something erupt inside of me. I couldn't make sense of it, but I was carried by it like an unstoppable destructive tide, tears spilling from my eyes. I heard myself shouting. I saw his surprised face, but I could not stop. I didn't mean to shout but words were escaping my mouth at a volume I couldn't control. I sounded angry but it was more than that.

When we got home, I burst into the toilet, bladder once again burning and the whirlpool of emotions I still couldn't fathom gaining intensity. Collapsed on the bathroom floor, I sobbed at a loss of what to do. I felt so alone and misunderstood. At some point the despair gave way to a steely resignation that some part of me tried to take comfort from knowing *'there is no point to anything'*. This moment in time had a profound impact on me and my partner. I'd reached a depth of despair that felt irreversible in some way. Like having been there, life would never be the same again.

Now I have a far better understanding of why I felt like this. It relates to those core safety threats I introduced you to at the start of this book (page 14). First was the mistrust and sense of betrayal I felt from my body. All the physical suffering and reactions to medications meant that I no longer trusted that I could rely on it or that it could withstand basic challenges like a couple of drinks on a night out. This created intense fear and unease, which affected my sense of social safety (Chapter 7 will explain the psychobiology of this further). It meant that I had this unshakeable feeling of 'otherness' for which I was desperately compensating, piling immense amounts of pressure on myself. These made up the second and third threats of disconnection and self-blame.

My partner's comment triggered all these emotions to rise and break through the surface. It was the contrast of how easily he had assimilated and how hard I had tried to and failed. I was struck by the grief of all that had changed. The deep longing for a body I could trust. For the ability to inhabit the world as though I belonged in it again. And to be relieved from the disturbing, visceral sense that I was a broken, faulty mess of no significance to anyone, despite how hard I tried.

This would not be the last time I felt intensely uncomfortable for all these reasons, but it was the last time I felt so convinced there was no point. And that is because I was able to process some of these feelings. To better know, feel and eventually resolve them. This has allowed me to trust my body again and even feel compassion if I have the slightest of bladder twinges, which are few and far between and never last longer than minutes. It has meant that I regard my bladder as a barometer of my needs rather than a tyrannical betrayer. Working through difficult emotions and moments like this has helped me to make peace with who I am now. Different to before but not deficient. Wiser and more compassionate. Processing what came up that night meant that I didn't run away from new attempts to socialize or find new friends and *that* meant that I once again could experience a sense of belonging.

In this chapter, we'll explore why your own emotional experiences aren't always clear to you and how when they do become clearer, you may find yourself responding in ways that don't serve you. This chapter will contextualize reactive responses to emotions by considering the biological basis of them, clarifying why emotions and symptoms often coincide and reducing self-blame. It was not the alcohol that made my bladder burn that night.

You'll learn how to make your body feel safe when experiencing intense emotions so that they don't contribute to threat mode and how to befriend your emotions so that experiences of difficult emotions can feel equalizing – even empowering. Befriending emotions follows three principles: acknowledgement, expression and soothing. You don't always need to exercise all three.

Emotions: physical events in the body

Emotions are natural experiences with physical footprints in the body that span your brain, nervous system, organs and somatic senses. The experience of emotions is highly individual. If your vitals were monitored and your brain scanned whilst feeling anxious, it might look physiologically very different to mine if I were monitored. There aren't universal physiological signatures for emotions. That's because emotions are the result of multiple things happening at once. Your brain integrates a multitude of potentially

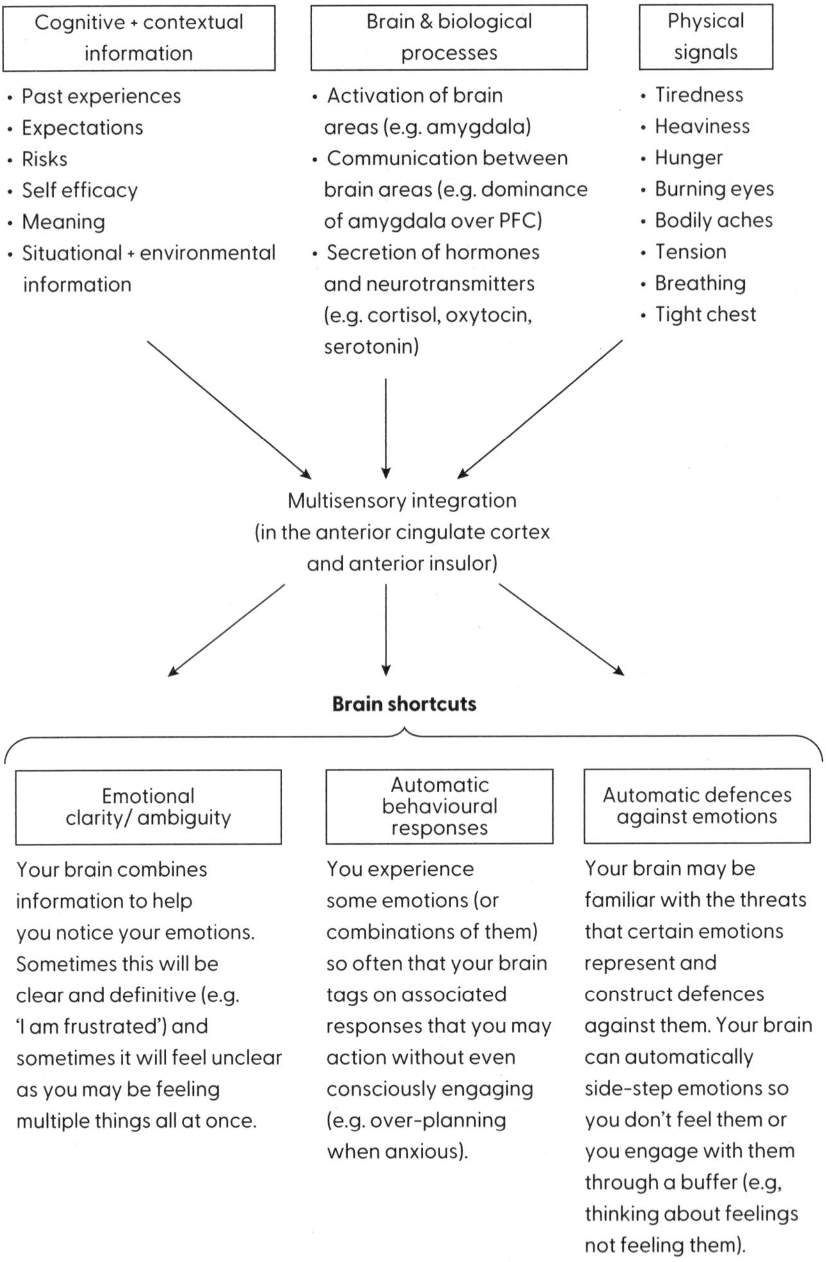

Cognitive + contextual information	Brain & biological processes	Physical signals
• Past experiences • Expectations • Risks • Self efficacy • Meaning • Situational + environmental information	• Activation of brain areas (e.g. amygdala) • Communication between brain areas (e.g. dominance of amygdala over PFC) • Secretion of hormones and neurotransmitters (e.g. cortisol, oxytocin, serotonin)	• Tiredness • Heaviness • Hunger • Burning eyes • Bodily aches • Tension • Breathing • Tight chest

Multisensory integration
(in the anterior cingulate cortex and anterior insulor)

Brain shortcuts

Emotional clarity/ ambiguity	Automatic behavioural responses	Automatic defences against emotions
Your brain combines information to help you notice your emotions. Sometimes this will be clear and definitive (e.g. 'I am frustrated') and sometimes it will feel unclear as you may be feeling multiple things all at once.	You experience some emotions (or combinations of them) so often that your brain tags on associated responses that you may action without even consciously engaging (e.g. over-planning when anxious).	Your brain may be familiar with the threats that certain emotions represent and construct defences against them. Your brain can automatically side-step emotions so you don't feel them or you engage with them through a buffer (e.g, thinking about feelings not feeling them).

Figure 19: How your body and brain integrate multimodal information to produce emotional experiences and automatic responses to emotions.

very different physiological processes (e.g. heart rate, shifts in dopamine levels, increased reactivity to adrenaline etc.), brain activity, sensory and psychological experiences (Figure 19). This is a complex calculation your brain computes to figure out what emotion/s you are feeling. Much of this 'calculating' takes place in the ACC and the anterior insula.* Sometimes, when there are lots of multi-sensory data and thought processes, the calculation gets jumbled, making it hard to get clarity on what you are feeling emotionally.

You likely have experienced moments of being caught between 'head' and 'heart'. Your 'thinking brain' is telling you one thing (cognitive processes in Figure 19), but you *feel* differently. This is reflective of frictions between activation in different brain regions. Dorsal brain regions are more analytical and cognitively sophisticated so that you can work things out and think creatively ('thinking brain'). Ventral regions are areas of your brain that house many of the emotion-centred brain structures ('emotional brain'). Generally, your brain is good at integrating information, but sometimes the contrast feels too big. For example, if you feel utterly overwhelmed or anxious, you may feel that you need to take the day off work (ventral region activity). And yet your thinking brain (dorsal) may be concerned with the impact of doing that, making you unsure what you should listen to.

Sometimes your 'thinking brain' is overriding important emotional and physiological experiences that you need to acknowledge (we'll explore later). Other times, your 'emotional brain' is dominating (remember amygdala hijack, page 49) and inhibiting your ability to see things with objectivity. This is a phenomenon briefly mentioned in Chapter 3: emotional reasoning. You feel anxious, so you assume you'll feel out of place if you meet up with friends. You feel guilty, so you offer to over-extend yourself. You feel angry, so the question you are asked seems provoking and rude.

There is an additional layer to emotional reasoning when you

---

* You may remember these brain areas in the role they play in pain processing.

have physical symptoms. Your brain makes sense of what emotions you are experiencing, partly by how you are physically feeling (Figure 19). Physical discomfort can send erroneous signals, that can intensify emotions or confuse the clarity of emotional experiences. To make sense of this, your dorsal (thinking) regions will look at the data it has (what is happening, what has just happened, what sensations you're feeling) and will propose reasons for why you feel as you do. Sometimes this will be spot on and other times not so much. For example, you may conclude you feel unsociable because you're too unwell in moments when you could still benefit from socializing.

Emotions have an evolutionary function of motivating behaviour to keep you safe. Feeling fear, motivates you to be on guard. Evolutionarily this would prevent you being eaten by a predator. Feeling guilt, motivates prosocial behaviour. Evolutionarily this would keep you in favour with your tribe. In modern-day life, emotions have similar functions, but with different threats and more evolved pursuits they can get confusing. Because of this primary motivational function, the brain often creates 'shortcuts' (Figure 19), so that a particular emotion will elicit an automatic reaction in the body and/or behaviourally. Feeling uncertainty may automatically compel you to research.

When your brain's calculations are accurate enough, you get a good sense of how you feel, why and how to respond appropriately. However, with just a few data points slightly off, your brain can come up with appraisals and responses that don't serve you (as you have seen in symptom spirals).

Jack's story

One of my clients, Jack, realized his brain had miscalculated, when he left his job because of how stressed he felt at work because of his health. He'd been feeling uncomfortable for a while because he was always aware of deadlines that he *may* miss or that his colleagues *may* have to 'pick up the slack' if he had to excuse himself due to symptoms. So, he decided to quit.

One glum autumn day, I blinked as I heard that he'd quit his job a while back. His brow was furrowed as he shared that he'd made a terrible mistake. It had been some months since quitting. The time that had passed clarified to him just how much he enjoyed his job. Since he'd left, the uncomfortable feelings he'd been having at work were still there. His voice broke as he explained that he'd assumed he was experiencing extra anxiety because his work wasn't right for him, given his diagnosis of MS. Although his symptoms weren't severe and he was able to complete his work, when a colleague approached his desk his heart would race and he'd immediately feel like his physical health was being compromised.

As we explored things, it became clear that his brain had been trying to make sense of the additional physical sensations he was getting when he felt this anticipatory anxiety. It had concluded that as this happened mainly in work, work was the problem. More specifically work must be bad for him.

Leaving his job had shown him that he still experienced the physical spikes of discomfort intermingled with anxiousness. It could happen with his partner or even his family. He realized his body generally felt unsafe and it was making him believe that the context in which he was in was the unsafe thing.

As you may imagine, it was a huge blow to realize he had let something go that was very meaningful to him and a source of security. While there was initially a lot of self-blame, that started to recede as Jack discovered something else: the power of interoceptive awareness.

Making emotions safer

You were introduced to how crucial interoceptive awareness is for detecting your body's physical needs and restoring balance (homeostasis). As emotions are physiological events in the body, your interoceptive awareness also affects your emotional awareness and consequent ability to process your emotions (Figure 20).

Since quitting his job, Jack had been building interoceptive awareness and was now able to notice that he'd been interpreting his heightened heartbeat, minor temperature changes and increased bodily tension as a sign that his body was unsafe in the context he was in. With this increased interoceptive awareness he was experiencing sensations differently. He could more readily link those subtle (and sometimes not so subtle) bodily cues with feeling anxious. He had also observed that these feelings became more likely whenever there was an expectation on him to perform. Be it a task that others could observe, like deciding what to eat on a menu when out with friends, or something where he had responsibility to act, like a job. These observations helped him see that expectations made his body react as though threatened because he was concerned his MS meant he couldn't meet them. We'll unpack concerns like this in Chapter 7, but for now let's stay with the significant shift that came from that increased interoceptive awareness.

When you are impacted by illness/trauma, the body tries to keep you safe by going into threat-detecting mode which creates a ripple effect throughout the nervous system and can contribute to dysregulation of your regulatory systems. This can increase pain, gut issues, fatigue, brain fog and impair immune functioning.

Building interoceptive awareness is a powerful antidote to threat mode on two levels:

1. **Emotion regulation**: Research conclusively shows that when you have high interoceptive awareness, you are more able to reduce the intensity of uncomfortable or intense emotions.[1,2] This ability is called 'emotion regulation'. Emotions are with you but not completely on top of you. From this position, in time, those emotions can healthily fade. The more regulated your emotional state, the more easily your body steps out of threat mode.

2. **Bodily regulation**: Enhancing your interoceptive awareness allows you to attend to your experience of bodily signals with clarity, less emotional reactivity and spiralling thoughts.[3,4,5] This skill automatically interrupts a multitude of psychobiological loops that would perpetuate threat mode. Studies show that people with chronic conditions who have more interoceptive awareness have less severe and frequent symptoms.[6]

Building interoceptive awareness enhances your ACC and anterior insula's ability to sort out the many signals they receive (Figure 19) and integrate them with more accuracy. It trains your brain to better know and handle intense experiences. Without this, it could continue knee-jerk and heavy-handed responses contributing to further emotional and physical dysregulation.

Emotional awareness

In Chapter 4, you were introduced to the nervous system barometer and how to notice the experience of physical and emotional experiences side by side. By practising this, already you have been improving your brain's ability to integrate signals less reactively. Practising this also helps you identify *how* you experience different emotions in your body. How emotions are felt in the body is not the same for everyone, but there are commonalities which have been illustrated in the largest 'emotion mapping' study to date. This study found that people tend to feel anxiety as warmth in the chest and gut. In contrast, during sadness there is decreased sensation in the limb areas.[7]

When working with clients, I usually start with exercises that help to physically inhabit the body and build interoceptive awareness, with focus on the sensory experience. That means homing in on the variety, quality and dynamics of physical experiences, whilst noticing how that corresponds with emotions. To use Jack as an example, this would mean exploring how he felt his heartbeat, the strength of beats, how his chest felt around that, what happened in his shoulders and breathing, any temperature shifts and where and how he felt that, etc. We would observe how all of this corresponded with his emotional experience of anxiety and anything else, but we wouldn't bring emotions centre stage in the initial phases.

As this developed, I would then start to bring emotional awareness to the forefront. Bringing emotions centre stage means that we keep turning towards whatever sense there is of emotion/s and noticing what comes *with* that experientially. Often thoughts come in, in which case we redirect back to the body gently.

For Jack, that would have involved exploring the experience of anxiety. How did he know he was anxious? What was happening most strongly to tell him he was anxious? Jack would have pointed to the tight chest and heart rate that felt inextricable from anxiety, but also the sense of being frozen in bodily tension. With that there was the racing mind full of sentiments that something needed to change. As we spent time observing this, the experience of anxiety merged with guilt and self-blame. This was followed by intense fear and an urge to fix. More physical symptoms accompanied the intolerability of these emotions. You can see how shifting the metaphorical angle could bring some aspects of the experience into closer view and clarity.

Whilst I generally start building interoceptive awareness with a focus on the physical experience (using the nervous system barometer), how long we spend there, and what we do to increase emotional awareness, depends on several things. Namely, where you are on the emotion identification spectrum (Figure 20).

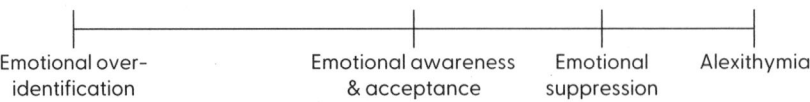

Figure 20: The emotion identification spectrum – a spectrum of the different ways people can identify with and relate to their emotions.

Your relationship with your emotions

Do you know how you feel? And do you know how you know?

By exploring this with my clients, I have come to recognize a variety of relationships with emotions along a continuum (Figure 20). On one end there is emotional 'over-identification'. Here the volume of emotions is turned right up and it's hard to see anything without the taint of the mood state. Individuals here have high levels of emotional reasoning and find it hard to listen to the dorsal (thinking) brain. What we are aiming for is somewhere along the continuum towards the middle: emotional awareness and acceptance. We'll come back to this.

At the opposite end of the continuum is emotional suppression. In Chapter 3, we considered the various ways this can manifest. Emotional suppressors are more likely to report feeling OK or fine when things are very stressful. At the furthest end of this continuum is alexithymia. Alexithymia describes reduced awareness of emotions and difficulties in describing them. It can be a personality trait, or a state brought on by stress, trauma or mental illness. Although alexithymia can be someone's default personality characteristic or associated with neurodivergence, like autism (although not a universal trait of autism), it is something that is changeable, as are all the ways of relating to your emotions. Approaches that nurture a person's ability, intention and acceptability of attending to how they feel emotionally can increase their emotional insight and regulation.[8,9]

For those with less emotional awareness, spending time building up sensory-led interoceptive awareness (or body awareness), as described in Chapter 4, will create a foundation for increasing emotional clarity.

Spotting and labelling emotions can help further with this. Using the 'feelings wheel' tool developed by Dr Gloria Willcox[10] can help increase familiarity of your emotional experiences (Figure 21).

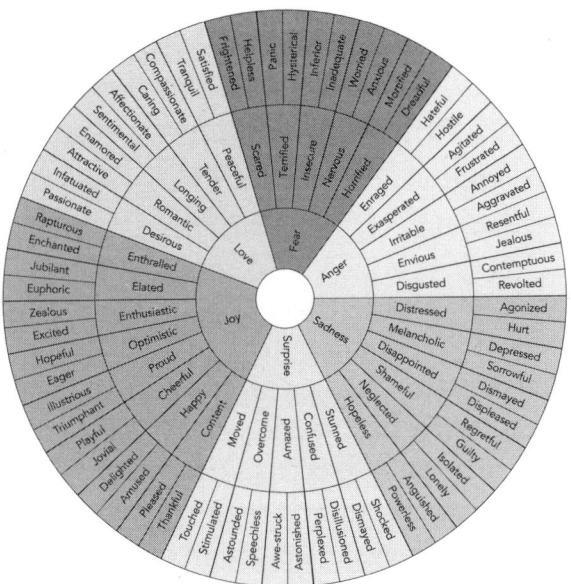

Figure 21: Feelings wheel.

The practice:

1. Note that you are having an emotional experience (of any kind) and rate your clarity on how you feel (0 not at all, 10 completely).
2. Use the emotion wheel, starting with the middle to identify the broad emotion.
3. Span to the outer circle to see what specific emotions you identify with on any level (cognitively, emotionally or somatically).
4. Pause on each emotion you identify with to see if you can feel it in your body.
5. Re-rate how much clarity you have on how you feel.

If none of the words on the wheel seem to fit, this is an exciting learning opportunity for your ACC and anterior insula. You don't need clarity, just curiosity. Note which words feel the closest and pay close attention to how your body feels. Just by turning towards this ambiguous emotional experience you've helped your brain to reduce automatic threat appraisals and responses that may have otherwise been initiated. This trains your brain to greet your emotions. Over time your brain learns that difficult emotions are safe, reducing physiological stress reactions to them.[11] That is powerful.

Adjusting the volume of emotions

When you have less emotional awareness or a tendency towards suppression, interoceptive awareness practices help you to increase the 'volume' of your emotions. That means increasing the intensity and clarity of emotional experiences. Professor of psychiatry Dan Siegel developed the concept of the 'window of tolerance' for emotion regulation. When you experience emotions within your window of tolerance, your body can respond optimally to the distress (Figure 22). You can access your rational brain and function socially.

When you are below your window of tolerance, your bodily systems are in a state of 'hypoarousal' akin to the deactivated/shut down mode of the nervous system barometer. This contributes to the cumulation of stress in the body (allostatic load). Therefore, we want to increase the volume of your emotional experience so that you can psychologically and physiologically regulate.

Debra's story

My client Debra came to me because she was having repeated urinary tract infections every one to three months. She'd used every medical treatment but to no avail. A key focus for our therapy was to increase her access to her emotions, building tolerance and acceptance. It was not easy work and there were many sessions where she would ask me indignantly, 'Why are we doing this again?'

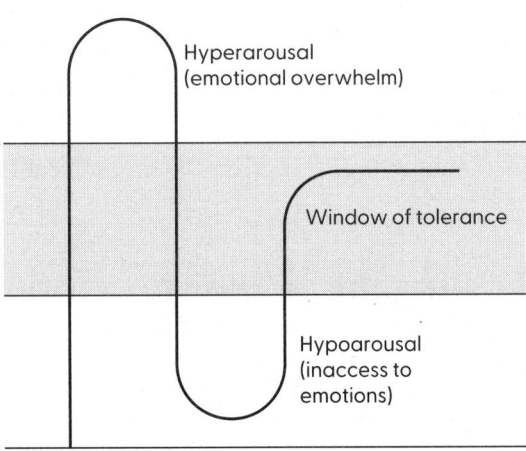

The line depicts potential 'tolerance zones' for emotional experiences often correlating with physiological arousal.

Hypoarousal is where there is a lack of emotional arousal or engagement, whereas hyperarousal is where emotions are experienced as overwhelming.

The middle window of tolerance is the target zone for accessing emotions but not becoming overwhelmed by them. This zone is also where your body is most able to physiologically regulate.

Figure 22: Emotional window of tolerance.

Sometimes the question was genuine because feeling the feelings hurt, but other times it was rhetorical. She could see what shifted when she chose to feel. There was an access to herself, her values and the life that she wanted, when she felt what had previously been pushed down. In a way that was hard for her to articulate, she felt alive and connected. She feared herself less. The sense that there was a big, destructive monster inside was fading. And with that fade, she reflected twelve months later, she had not had one urinary tract infection. Although counterintuitive, bringing emotions to the surface makes your body more able to heal because it alleviates the burden of suppression. Suppression is an active physiological process that requires coordination between the brain and regulatory systems.[12,13]

Turning up the volume on your emotions, so you are hearing more from them, is a precarious process. You need to be able to swiftly adjust the volume down when it becomes a bit too loud (emotionally intense), as can often happen when we're making space to feel. This is a skill too. If you've rarely had intense emotions, suddenly being faced with the challenge of reducing that intensity can make you question your ability to do so. That's why it is important to develop the skills of dynamic volume shifting: feeling a little bit more and then allowing those feelings to be soothed or dissipated. We'll come to that in a moment.

Those who experience emotions loudly and intensely (on the left side of the emotion identification continuum) will benefit from practices that focus on reducing the intensity (volume) of emotions. When emotions are too intense you are pushed up and out of this window of tolerance in a state of hyperarousal (Figure 22). This is overwhelming and would put you in the activated state on the nervous system barometer.

Adjusting the volume of emotions in acute moments of overwhelm generally involves working directly with the body to regulate. Breathing practices, engaging your senses, and grounding can all help you turn down the volume on intense activation in the emotion regions of your brain.

Feeling emotions calmly*

1. As you become aware that you are feeling emotions too intensely for comfort, picture that high activation in the middle part of your brain. Use this to detach from your thought stream and bring your awareness to your body.
2. Notice how your whole body feels. Note areas of tension and any urges you have to move or react. Come to your breath.

---

* Audio guidance available www.healthpsychologist.co.uk/itsallinyourbody

3. Slow your breathing down, so that both the in and out breath are gradual, deep and long. Imagine rationing your breath bit by bit. As you breathe, transport your breath all the way down to your stomach. As you breathe in, your belly expands out and as you exhale your belly comes back in. See if you can extend your exhale longer than your in-breath. This activates your parasympathetic nervous system, helping your ANS to calm down your brain and body.
4. When emotions feel less intense, decide if you want to turn towards whatever got you emotionally activated and work with it in some way, or whether you will do something else to allow you to regulate further. This is what you may consider to be 'distraction' but I often call 'tethering'.

Accepting your feelings

You don't always need an intervention to reduce emotional distress or discomfort. Difficult or unpleasant emotions are not bad for your body if you can experience them within your window of tolerance. It might sound odd, but being able to feel 'bad' in your window of tolerance is *good* for your health. The alternative is always having to feel 'good', for positive emotions to be in your window of tolerance. Being able to feel OK about feeling sad or anxious can be immensely liberating. This is emotional acceptance – being at peace with emotions that aren't naturally pleasant.

'Acceptance' is a tricky word as you may immediately equate it with resignation. But resignation is passive. It is a giving up. Acceptance is a fierce and intentional permission, flexible and fluid. Summed up in a sentence, emotional acceptance is you saying and believing 'this is how I feel, *for now*'. There is no judgement or resistance but there is a recognition that it won't remain the same. With that, there may also be knowledge of what scope you have to change things without the urgency to enact it *now*. This reduces the pressure and fear that can arise from difficult feelings, to escape them.

After my outburst on that night, I felt a lot of shame and guilt. I felt it was an over-reaction, and my poor partner must think I was unstable. In the following days, I was subdued, skulking around our flat, with sunken eyes and bowed head. The feelings that had come to the surface that night still gnawed at me but now they were weighed with shame. It was in the way I moved, slow and sloping. As my loving partner gently explored my feelings with me, helped me to understand them, this changed. Although the sense of grief was still there, the shame dissipated. My relationship with my grief was different now. It was beside me, not dragging behind me. Although it remained with me for a while, I had the fizz of determination in my gut, my head lifted, directed ahead and not down, my eyes to the horizon. My shoulders were not quite so sloped, and I now moved with purpose. Beside me, the grief was no longer pulling me back. 'This is how I feel, *for now*.'

Interoceptive practices create foundations for building that flexible curiosity towards emotions. To help your logical brain accept that feeling emotion is OK and doesn't need to be fixed, you may need to address your automatic defences against emotions.

Recognizing resistance

Powerlessness is one of those emotions that is particularly threatening to your sense of safety and thematic in this book. Earlier, I referenced the automatic shortcuts your brain generates to help you escape overwhelming emotions like powerlessness. Resistance to feeling emotions can be one of these shortcuts.

Internal family systems therapy (IFS) distinguishes the experience of emotions that make you feel vulnerable and powerless from the resistance that can come with feeling these emotions.[14] The former experience is attributed to a specific 'exile' part of you, that has not been allowed to acknowledge or process emotions. The other 'protector' parts have developed to try and prevent you from feeling these difficult emotions because they have been overwhelming and destabilizing, deemed useless.

One of these protector parts is called the 'manager'. This is an extremely 'thinky' part, that likes ration, logic and reason. When in managerial mode, there may be more activation in the dorsal brain regions. It has a very effective and, on some level, comforting way of minimizing difficult emotions. It can also go into overdrive to prevent future instances of distress. It does this through planning and analysing. This creates a high cognitive load. Unfortunately, a high cognitive load can overtax the regulatory systems,[15] negatively impacting your health. You may recall that high volume cognitive processing demands a lot of energy and resource from your body and increases glutamate. Increased demand when physically under-resourced creates fatigue, brain fog, pain, headaches and more. Your brain will continue to deem this a worthwhile trade-off when it is fearful of being with emotions, so it is important to make emotions feel safer.

Negotiating emotions with resistant parts*

This journaling exercise is intended to help you separate your manager part from your exile, whilst having you (your wiser, adult self) become the mediator between the two. This involves some mental imagery work, but if you find it hard to visualize, you can use the guidance purely as narrative journaling prompts.

1. Close your eyes and picture yourself at a table. You are joined by your manager (analytical) and your exile (emotional). Take a moment to visualize how your manager appears, their manner, tone and expression. Do the same for your exile. How do they relate to each other? Is the exile happy to defer to the manager or does it feel closed down? How does the manager regard the exile?

---

* Audio guidance available www.healthpsychologist.co.uk/itsallinyourbody

2. Next, you're going to negotiate with the manager that you would like to make space to acknowledge the exile. You can put the case to the manager with logic (it likes that), referring to passages from this book to make your case about why this is important for your healing goals. You are not trying to strong-arm the manager – it can be very stubborn. You want to bring it along with you.
3. When it allows a bit of space to turn towards the exile, this is your chance to be open and explorative but not analytical. You are trying to understand this part not to fix or get rid of it. Treat it as though you have a small child that is experiencing feelings it doesn't know how to handle and you just want to reassure it that that's OK. You are there to let it know, whatever is there, you want to hear.

For some this feels very wishy-washy. For others it feels immensely cathartic straight away. It can be a hard practice to do on your own, but when you are able to it can be incredibly powerful. Try it out in different mood states.

Cherie's story

One of my clients, Cherie, had been dealing with severe anxiety for a long time, as well as a lot of physical symptoms including chronic pain. Her emotional experience confused her. Her anxiety felt logical – there were things that *could* go wrong – and yet in some situations she remained stoic and calm in a way that felt at odds with her anxiety.

We started doing IFS parts work because we recognized that she had not been allowed to feel vulnerable emotions that did not make sense or were not 'fixable'. The unacceptability of emotions was linked with her pain. 'Unfixable' emotions and pain snapped the manager into action, often exacerbating pain.

One session, we explored through parts work what it had been like to experience specific pain episodes. She was surprised that connecting with her exile resulted in tears and previously un-accessed sadness and sense of abandonment. We explored gently, asking the manager to 'sit' to one side so we could comfort this exile and hear a little more. At the end of the session I asked, 'How does that exile feel now?' Cherie told me that it felt reassured and comforted that it was not alone and was finally getting the recognition of pain it had never had before. She was confused because *she* was all too aware of the pain she'd been feeling. How could a part of her exist that felt on its own?

Neuroscience can partly explain this. The brain consists of multiple neural networks responsible for different functions and behaviours. These networks can operate semi-independently, leading to varied responses in different contexts. This neural architecture supports the idea of distinct 'parts' within the mind. The medial prefrontal cortex (mPFC) has a major role in self-referential thinking, emotion regulation and pain processing. Significantly it also has a role in processing social rejection and the overlap with physical pain.

When Cherie experienced pain, the mPFC may well have established a neural network that was characterized by a sense of isolation and helplessness in relation to pain. Because her default emotional coping involved suppressing such feelings, activity here may have been deactivated as has been observed before in experiences of self-abandonment.[16] This may explain why it felt a part of her was being acknowledged for the first time when she intentionally turned towards these emotions using parts work. This kind of parts work elicits compassion and studies demonstrate that eliciting compassion can increase activation of the mPFC.[17] Parts work was helping her change her brain processing as well as her psychological and physical experience.

Cost of constant distraction

If one defence against emotions is this managerial 'thinky' mode, another is what is called in IFS therapy, your 'firefighter' part.

While the manager is focussed on prevention of potential negative feelings, the firefighter swiftly steps in when negative feelings become overwhelmingly present. Distraction is a common tool for the firefighter. It can be quite astonishing to see this part in action.

Here is an example from therapy:

I smile at my client, with anticipation. This is the session we'd agreed to start some trauma processing (using EMDR). I set up for processing by orienting the client to the memory we've chosen to process, inviting them to allow their brain to go anywhere intuitively. Like a process of free-association. When I check in moments later, I am greeted by the firefighter.

'Nothing.' A shrug. Laissez-faire. Maybe an apology. Or a throw-up of hands, 'What can you do?'

I'm fond of the firefighter part. It does its job so well. I explore with it a little, 'Nothing came up at all?' I ask whether they felt *anything*, when 'nothing' came up. Where did the mind go? Funnily enough, often when I ask this, it seems the mind did go somewhere of significance, so we follow that. Other times thoughts are seemingly unrelated (e.g. to-do list).

It will take a few more rounds of 'nothing' before I begin to address that firefighter part directly. When I do, I'm exploring with it what it fears will happen if my client fully engages in the emotion of the memory. This is often when we get somewhere.

'I'll be a mess for the rest of the day.'

'It's not fair to my mum.'

'It's embarrassing.'

Whatever comes up, we work with compassionately, processing the resistance to being with emotion. This makes emotion safer.

From a neuroscience perspective, the firefighter is the learnt brain responses to avoiding emotional overwhelm by utilizing distraction. Your PFC detects that unpleasant activation in the limbic system and decides to divert your attention away. This is generally an automated subconscious process. In addition, your Default Mode Network (page 155) can activate in response to emotional distress, making your mind wander to unrelated thoughts. These processes can act on dopamine reward systems which positively reinforce you for distracting yourself. A good example of this is picking up your phone every time you are bored, impatient or anxious. Because it is so effective it keeps you using that strategy and quickly becomes habitual as neural pathways in the basal ganglia (area of your brain involved in habit formation) are strengthened every time you distract yourself from uncomfortable emotions.

In the short term, these ways of coping can be relieving, but long term they can make you avoid difficult emotions that need to be addressed. This may make it hard to have reparative conversations with others, for fear of it being too upsetting. You may feel powerless to your devices and quick fixes like binge-eating or pacifying TV. These effects of emotional avoidance can directly impact your health through dysregulation of your regulatory systems and increased allostatic load.

Emotional avoidance also can prevent stressful and traumatic events from being adaptively integrated by your brain and filed away as past experiences. This can keep you emotionally and physically reactive. In the context of PTSD and trauma, avoidance of trauma-related thoughts and feelings changes the memory and emotion processing brain structure, the hippocampus. Avoidance and changed hippocampal function and structure is associated with more withdrawal and mood difficulties.[18,19,20] Whether or not you have PTSD, repeated emotional avoidance (distraction) impacts mood and health.[21,22,23]

When distraction works

Sometimes distraction can be an effective emotion regulation strategy. When you don't have mental or physical capacity to be with your feelings, it is OK to defer this. Coming out of surgery or at the start of a break-up, sometimes it is too raw to sit with and that's OK. You can lean into the auto-protection mode your brain offers. Having awareness and intention allows you to come back round to the feelings, when you have capacity.

Expressing yourself

As you start to become more aware of how you feel, it can be hard to simply 'sit' with it. For many of my patients, there aren't quick fixes to difficult emotions. They are simply natural responses to not being able to do things as you would like. Or to feeling physically unwell. Or to being treated poorly by others when you are already vulnerable and depleted.

Expressing how you feel is healing even when it is not heard by others. We'll consider expressing yourself to others more centrally in Chapter 7. In this section, we're focussing on 'internal expression': emotionally expressing for yourself. Things like writing letters you'll never send, shouting out loud, punching a pillow or journaling. All of these are emotion expression options.

'Expressive writing' is a practice that involves writing for fifteen to twenty minutes about emotional, stressful or traumatic events to express related feelings and thoughts. Decades of research have shown that it can improve physical and mental health outcomes for those with and without physical or mental health diagnoses. Expressive writing can directly benefit multiple regulatory systems, with documented physiological benefits including improved blood pressure, lung function, immune system function and liver function.[24] A 2024 comprehensive meta-analysis looked at the results of thirty-four studies including over 4,000 women with breast cancer and found that expressive writing improved fatigue and meant that patients were more able to do their day-to-day activities like walking, household tasks or general social activities.[25] Interestingly, these improvements happened without changing anxiety or depression, reflecting how expression of emotion can directly interact with your biology to improve health. Other studies with other groups have found expressive writing can also significantly improve mood outcomes including depression and anxiety.[26] Writing with shorter intervals (one to three days) between expressive writing tends to have more of an effect than doing it every four to seven days or longer.

Expressive writing

Pick a time you will sit down to write for fifteen to twenty minutes every two to three days.

Write your deepest thoughts and feelings about difficult issues facing you now or from the past. It does not matter which you choose. You can choose differently each time you write.

When writing, try and let go of trying to make sense of the experience or of being reasonable and fair. This is your time to allow any feelings or thoughts to come up. You can be repetitive, inarticulate, with bad grammar and wrong spelling. All that matters is you allow yourself to write.

Set a timer and continue until your time is up.

You may like to check in with your body after doing this using the nervous system barometer.

The art of savouring

Emotional regulation is not just about learning to be with the difficult emotions. It's about making space to feel emotions you like to feel too. Threatened brains and nervous systems prioritize threat-salient information, so it's important to counterbalance intentionally by turning towards and embracing positive and even neutral emotional experiences. A practice I incorporate with all of my clients early on is a polyvagal informed practice called 'savouring' by trauma therapist Deb Dana.[27]

> **Savouring**
>
> Each day, intentionally pay attention to and lean into positive or neutral emotional experiences for thirty to sixty seconds. This might be noticing the absence of pain and the peace around that, staying with that experience for just thirty seconds or so. Or really savouring that first sip of hot coffee, cosy in your jumper on your couch. There is no minimum bar for pleasure or appreciation. Being present with a 2/10 pleasure maximizes the benefit of it. It's only a bonus when you come across a 10/10.

Learning to trust yourself (and body) again

On the night when my emotions plumed to the surface, I initially just wanted to escape the intensity of what I was feeling. It was all so painful and overwhelming. It was only on reflection that I could conceptualize it as grief: a deep longing for attachment that had been jeopardized by becoming ill. Jeopardized because I often felt so alone in my experience and suffering. That night, no one could see the frantic paddling that was happening just under the surface, and it felt like no one cared to know. When I'd gone to therapy, as clear as I'd tried to be, my specific requests for help had gone unheard. All of this eroded my trust in my own ability and in the cooperation and support of others. Navigating a world that feels hostile, with no confidence in your own armour, understandably feels too much.

Grief is a common experience when your life has changed in a direction you didn't choose. It is an 'unfixable feeling' as you can't rationalize it away or try and perceive things differently. It is there because you are dealing with a difficult reality. But far from 'unfixable' meaning it won't ever feel bearable, unfixable perhaps can be your invitation to acknowledge your feelings.

In this chapter we've covered:

- The physiological nature of emotions and underlying biological processes
- The spectrum of relationships you may have with your emotions
- How to start developing emotional awareness and adjust the intensity of your emotional experiences
- What resisting feelings does biologically, why this happens and how to make space for and accept emotions
- Healthy options for emotional expression.

Hopefully this chapter has given you an understanding of just how healing it can be to acknowledge feelings. With my clients, I marvel at how transformative it is to intentionally make space to recognize that 'exile' part without trying to fix it. I will ask my clients, 'How do you feel towards this part of you?' and their answers often reflect one thing: compassion. When I ask how this exile part feels to be acknowledged they tell me it is a relief. This may be accompanied by beautiful imagery of them embracing their past selves or sitting side by side in solidarity. Acknowledging feelings without trying to fix them is an important part of regaining trust in your body and in yourself. And, of course, trust is a key foundation of any friendship.

CHAPTER 6

Thinking yourself better or thinking yourself sick?

Before I was able to emotionally process, as discussed in the last chapter, there was something huge that had had to change first. My relationship with my thoughts.

One day back when I was still signed off work and staying with my dad, my self-care barely existent, I came downstairs where my dad had prepared two mats for us to practise mindfulness together. He had suggested it some days prior and, although resistant, I had agreed to try it. But my reluctance to try this, or anything else, was building again, my mood darkening and hope fading. Dark mood and outlook seemed to be my default now amongst the backdrop of bladder aches, burns, urgency and nightly migraine attacks.

I sat down to the instructions of Jon Kabat-Zinn, grandfather of mindfulness as is now practised in the Western world, telling us to breathe. To notice our bodies and to peel away from the thought streams and inhabit our experiences without trying to get a grip of what exactly that was. At one point during this meditation, he said, 'From the perspective of mindfulness, as long as you're breathing there is more right with you than wrong with you.' I still remember the jolt of annoyance and snarky, 'Yeah, that's alright for you to say, Jon, try having my bladder' thought. But then, something remarkable happened.

I *noticed* with clarity, both the anger and the thought. And in that noticing I felt a little silly and a little amused. I thought 'Ahh! *This* is mindfulness!' I had wandered into a different relationship with my experience. Rather than being consumed with more snarky thoughts and the usual feelings of injustice, I'd found an exit ramp. It wasn't a huge difference, but it was a definitive one. In contrast to the usual despairing thought loops, it felt a relief. It felt wiser, safer and less serious.

I continued practising and my ability to focus varied. So did the sense of wisdom and safety. But it had been there. And that kept me coming back. The more I practised, the more I could access that safe, non-reactive way of relating to my experience, including my bladder. When it spasmed, or jolted or threatened to burn for hours, I no longer automatically reacted with fear. And incredibly, my bladder pain started to subside. Even when I got twinges upon urinating, rather than sitting there trapped in mental calculations about how bad things were and may get, I could slow my breath, lessen my pounding heart and stand up from the toilet bowl, open to see what would happen next. Quite often I tentatively went about my business and there would be no follow-up pain. As my mental landscape became more spacious, my symptom spirals reduced. This approach drastically changed my relationship with my bladder and myself. I was on my own team and my body felt it.

This started to translate into more improvements in my physical symptoms. There were fewer migraines. Then no migraines. My vaginal PH balanced out. I stopped getting urinary tract infections. Although I wasn't 100% better, I felt confident enough to leave my job. This is what allowed me to make the decision to pack up my life in Leeds, move to London and start the master's in health psychology. Ultimately, this set in motion a whole chain of events that transformed my life for the better.

In this chapter, I'm going to clarify the role of thinking in healing. Moving away from 'it's all in your head' and reductive 'mind over matter' narratives, I'm going to explain the physicality of thinking and differentiate it from the attentional awareness and underlying beliefs you hold. This information aims to reduce any sense of self-blame for thoughts and pressure to correct your thinking. Instead, you're going to learn the principles of relating to your mental thought stream with neutrality, openness and curiosity and how this helps your body switch from threat mode to safety. With this foundation of accepting thoughts, you'll also learn strategies to work with the particularly difficult thoughts, and how to harness the healing powers of thinking.

Psychobiology of thoughts

Have you ever wondered where a thought came from? Or why you think something? The thinking mind is fascinating. Understanding a bit about the physiological basis of thinking can help you understand:

- How thinking can influence physical bodily experiences
- How thinking automatically elicits emotion even if you're not consciously aware of your thoughts
- How you can influence your thinking while not being accountable for the thoughts you have, or default thinking processes.

To consider all of this, let's break down the concept of 'thinking'. Thinking* involves three components: your thoughts, your attention and your beliefs. Your thoughts are patterns of electrical activity and chemical signalling in the brain depicted in Figure 23.

---

* Thinking is a complex neuropsychological topic. There are many more elements to thinking including memories, the different kinds of memory processing and the storing of knowledge. The three components depicted here are most relevant for the purpose of the chapter and working towards healing goals.

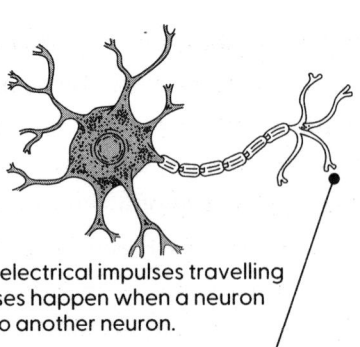

Thoughts are represented by electrical impulses travelling along neurons. These impulses happen when a neuron transmits a signal to another neuron.

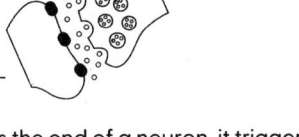

When the electrical impulse reaches the end of a neuron, it triggers the release of neurotransmitters (chemical messengers like dopamine) across the gap between neurons (synapses). This allows the signal to continue to the next neuron.

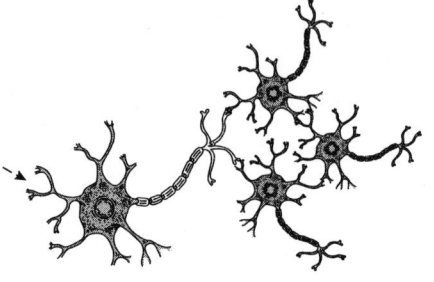

Thoughts emerge from patterns of neural activation across different brain areas.

Certain brain regions have a bigger role in directing thoughts.

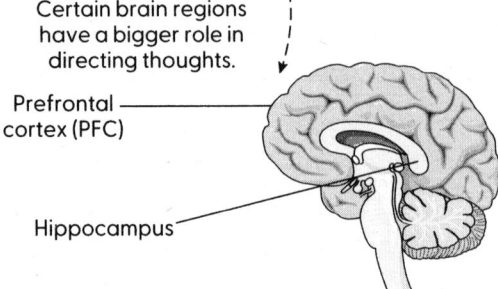

Prefrontal cortex (PFC)

Hippocampus

Figure 23: The biological basis of thinking.

As you think, your brain generates patterns of synchronized electrical activity. These patterns influence not only the specific thoughts you have but also your broader mental state. Here, 'mental state' refers to the different modes your mind operates in from cognitively alert states to more relaxed intuitive states (Table 9). A high volume of worried thoughts may create a heightened mental state, characterized by pressure to think and vigilant attentional processes. This occurs because both the content (what you are thinking) and cognitive style (how you are thinking) influence the type of brainwaves your brain produces. Brainwaves are distinct frequencies of electrical activity that correlate with different states of consciousness, shaping your mental state – whether calm, frantic, or engaged.

Brainwave patterns and the ways of thinking that they are

Table 9: Brainwave patterns and corresponding mental states		
Brainwave patterns	Mental state	When you experience this
Gamma waves (30–100Hz)	High level cognition & complex problem-solving	When learning and intensely processing information with heightened awareness, e.g. researching information about your health
Beta waves (12–30Hz)	Active thinking, problem-solving and focus	When deeply engaged in logical reasoning, work or conversation, e.g. experiencing discomfort or worrying about the future
Alpha waves (8–12Hz)	Calm awareness and creativity	When calm or in a reflective state, e.g. when daydreaming, meditating or feeling connected
Theta waves (4–8Hz)	Deep relaxation and intuition	When in a dreamy or hypnotic state, e.g. visualizing, creative flow or drifting to sleep

associated with, are shown in Table 9. Neuroscience research shows that the way you are thinking can both influence and be influenced by these different brainwave patterns (frequencies).[1] Bodily threat mode or high allostatic load can influence your brainwave patterns and, consequently, how you are thinking.[2] This is why it can be so hard to try and control your thoughts when you are highly anxious or when you feel deactivated and shut down. Your body is challenged, affecting your brain function and your psychological experience of thinking.

You can adapt your environment to help synchronize brainwaves to a calmer frequency.[3] When you go to a spa with low lighting and pink noise (e.g. nature sounds) this tends to elicit calm alpha brainwaves. Additionally, you can train your brain to process information in ways that promote brainwave patterns that are more regulating for mind and body.[4,5] The exercises coming up will help you to do this.

Your attention

If your thoughts are the content of what you think, underpinned by electrical signal transmissions, your attention is a neurological process that determines what elements of your experience are prioritized for you to attend to. Figure 24 illustrates the relationship between thoughts and attention. Attention is like a spotlight that can be trained internally on your emotional, physical or cognitive (thinking) experiences and/or externally to what is happening around you.

Different brain regions are involved in directing and honing attention. Some of them you will recognize from their role in emotion processing, the biological stress response, pain processing and trauma.

- **Prefrontal cortex (PFC)** – directs conscious attention and decision-making

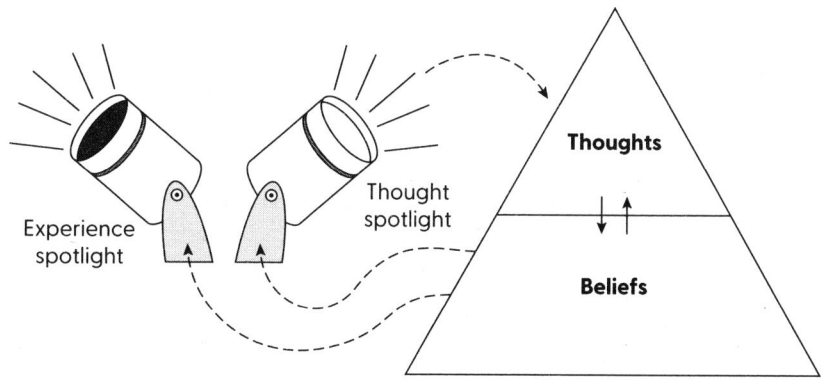

Figure 24: The relationship between attention, thoughts and beliefs.

- **Parietal cortex** – spatial awareness and shifts in attention
- **Thalamus** – filters sensory information (very important in the experience of physical symptoms)
- **Anterior cingulate cortex (ACC)** – regulates focus and detects conflicting information (e.g. when you notice a problem or are multitasking)
- **Basal ganglia** – helps sustain attention.

You also have neurotransmitters that regulate attention like dopamine, norepinephrine and acetylcholine. You may remember that these neurotransmitters are affected by the activity of your ANS and stress response. That means your attention can be enhanced or impeded by how threatened your body feels.

When you focus your attention on something, neurons in the relevant brain regions fire in synchrony, while brain areas that would process distractions are suppressed by inhibitory neurotransmitters. Imagine a musical conductor lifting their baton to elicit more from one part of the orchestra, while gesturing to keep other players quiet.

Brainwaves can also correspond to different types of attentional focus:

- Focussed attention involves fast active processing, underpinned by beta waves
- Relaxed awareness allows you to be calm but alert in an alpha wave state
- When distracted or experiencing low attentional focus, you may be in a theta wave state.

Your beliefs

Your thoughts and attention will be heavily influenced by your beliefs. While thoughts are momentary, beliefs are more deeply ingrained ideas. Thoughts that are repeated enough can create strong neural connections that form beliefs. Therefore, thoughts influence the development of beliefs, but once formed, beliefs heavily influence what you think and how you direct your attention. For example, if you have many experiences of being told your burnout is just you being lazy and not trying as hard as everyone else, you are going to start, at least in part, potentially believing that you are just not trying hard enough or that people will think you're lazy (or both). Then, when you are faced with disclosing a difficulty to a friend or colleague, these beliefs will direct your attention to notice all the subtleties in the interaction conveying that you're being judged. This will generate thoughts about what they thought of you, whether you said the right thing, etc. Figure 24 depicts the influence beliefs have over the directing of attentional spotlights and thoughts. Chapter 8 will consider beliefs in more detail.

Rethinking mind over matter

Mind-over-matter narratives tend to emphasize the importance of *what* you are thinking and the *control* you exercise over your thoughts. In my experience, in threatened, depleted bodies, these narratives can become disenfranchising and even harmful. They create pressure, which can itself change brain functioning. They also elevate attention on thoughts which, depending on the brainwave state you are in and the wider nervous system state, can create hypervigilance and more fear of thoughts. This fear and pressure create cognitive load (i.e. the amount of mental effort required to process information). High cognitive load can reduce your PFC's ability to emotionally regulate and can activate both the quick-fire (SAM system) and sustained (HPA axis) stress response, with the potential to impact physical symptoms and mood.[6]

Sam's story

My client Sam would tell me often, 'I know I shouldn't think that – I'm making it worse,' and she would find that her pain and bladder symptoms intensified. This wasn't because of *what* she was thinking. It was the perceived importance of these thoughts, her mental state and how much pressure she felt to think differently. We tested this hypothesis together one glum day, as she sat on her couch, discarded cup of tea to one side, and I on my swivel chair, the other side of Zoom. I asked her to close her eyes and see what thoughts came up. It was the usual thoughts about what her symptoms meant, how bad they may get and all the things she may not do well enough because of them. She told me with some urgency that her symptoms had intensified. I asked her to see if she could give herself permission to notice these thoughts, while not getting entangled in them – if she could come back to my guidance and to her body as she had been practising with the interoceptive practices.

I saw something subtle shift as she did this, my reassuring guidance now and again reminding her that thoughts were just electrical signals the brain uses to try and calculate. In that moment thoughts were neither true nor false. When she opened her eyes there was a spark. 'I've just realized how much my thoughts have been stressing me out! I've had a full-time job trying to correct them all the time!'

I asked her what had happened to her bladder pain as she'd sat with her thoughts. She blinked back. 'It's actually gone!'

I encouraged her to experiment over the coming weeks. In experimental condition one, thought control, she'd pick moments to notice difficult thoughts about symptoms and try hard to push them away or persuade herself they weren't true. In experimental condition two, thought permission, she'd allow difficult thoughts to be there as we'd done together. When I asked her how it had gone, she told me casually she'd abandoned the experiment a couple of days in, as the results were so clear. Realizing that she didn't have to control or monitor her thoughts released a huge amount of pressure, of which she physically felt the benefits. Her sleep was improved and she felt more present.

Sam's experience is reflected in research showing that trying to control or suppress thoughts can paradoxically lead to an increase in such thoughts.[7] It has been suggested that this strategy can cause the brain to assume the thoughts themselves are threats. To protect you from them, the brain amplifies their salience, bringing your attention to them when they arise. This can also activate nervous system pathways, potentially exacerbating physical symptoms and mood changes.

Before we explore working with your thoughts and attention to influence your mental state, let me reiterate: you are not to blame for your thoughts. You have thousands of thoughts a day, most of which you have not actively generated yourself and could not be held responsible for having. They are the product of neurons firing as your brain combines massive amounts of data and attempts to make sense of it and prioritize things that might be important. It stands to reason that thoughts that land with an emotional 'bang' are prioritized. This is why negative intrusive thoughts that randomly appear in your consciousness with some level of distress catch your attention. Although it can feel like you need to investigate, understand or counteract them, the most helpful thing you can do is to let them pass. Whether you are having intrusive thoughts about pushing someone off a platform, inflicting your symptoms on your friends or a montage of other unbearable scenarios, there's no need to fear. It does not make you a rotten person, just an alive one.

Updating your mental habits

How you interact with your thought stream, relate to your beliefs and harness (or not) your attention, will vary depending on the context, your mood, how you've been taught or shown to think and what is going on in your body. Mental habits are the ways that you process and relate to thoughts repeatedly. Mental habits are reinforced when they *seem* to work efficiently and effectively. Mental habits like worry and self-criticism get ingrained because they feel productive, so are reinforcing on some level, but they are disruptive long term.[8]

The first part of updating mental habits is noticing that you are engaging in them. In Chapter 3, you were introduced to different thinking patterns (page 128) that can perpetuate a sense of threat (e.g. foretelling the future, all-or-nothing thinking, mind-reading). Noticing these thinking patterns in action, builds something called metacognitive awareness. This is the ability to think about thinking. As you build metacognitive awareness, you improve connectivity between your PFC and other areas of the brain including your ACC, hippocampus and amygdala.[9,10,11] The increased connectivity improves your ability to focus your attention, consolidate memory (important for trauma processing) and regulate your emotions. It also has a direct effect on stress-related hormones and nervous system activity. All the practices included in this chapter will enhance your metacognitive awareness. You may like to refer back to page 25 to create specific stepping-stone goals related to this. What would you like to see change as you increase your ability to attend to your thoughts with more clarity and calm?

Thought-logging

Thought-logging is a strategy from CBT that involves capturing and writing down negative automatic thoughts that accompany difficult emotions and/or physical experiences. As well as building metacognitive awareness, it also helps you to shift long-standing negative beliefs that fuel ongoing negative thought patterns.[12] For example, '*My symptoms are going to get worse*' is an automatic negative thought that arises from a deeper belief system that you are not safe in your body or that you are doomed to suffer forever. When you notice how repetitive these negative automatic thoughts are, spotting the themes across them and the brain shortcuts in operation, you can start to regard them as they really are: mental events, not facts. As mental events they feel less distressing and are less physically activating.

Noticing thoughts

Over the next week, set the intention to notice the negative thoughts you have. Write them down when you can and classify them according to the thinking pattern they fall into. These thinking patterns were introduced in Chapter 3: fortune telling, emotional reasoning, all-or-nothing, mind reading and self-criticism.

You don't have to log every negative thought. Just a selection each day. At the end of the week, reflect on the themes of thoughts coming up and thinking patterns. Note any reflections you have. Explore the following questions:

- What is being filtered out and how does that shape how you feel?
- What good has come from these thoughts and thinking this way?
- How would you like to respond when you spot these kinds of thoughts in a way that will make you feel safer?

Situation	Thought	Thinking pattern, e.g. fortune telling, emotional reasoning, all-or-nothing, mind reading and self-criticism
e.g. organizing holiday	What if I ruin it for my partner by getting ill?	Self-critical, fortune telling

Mindfulness

Mindfulness, in its traditional context, is primarily a spiritual and philosophical practice aimed at increasing present-moment and self-awareness, and ultimately, enlightenment. In the twentieth century, mindfulness was secularly adapted and integrated into Western psychology practices. Jon Kabat-Zinn, a molecular biologist who studied under Buddhist teachers like Thích Nhất Hạnh and Seung Sahn, developed an eight-week programme called mindfulness-based stress reduction (MBSR), bringing mindfulness practice into the context of health and psychology. Since then, mindfulness has been adapted further in related therapies like mindfulness-based cognitive therapy (MBCT) and mindful-self compassion (MSC).

These approaches differ in their delivery of mindfulness, but the essence of the practices are the same. Mindfulness practice involves intentionally harnessing your awareness with an attitude of curiosity, compassion and non-judgement. The focus of your mindfulness practice may differ from practice to practice. In one practice you may pay attention to thoughts, in another to emotions or bodily sensations. In open mindful awareness you allow your attention to go to whatever naturally arises, with the intention of observing this rather than getting lost in more thoughts or analysis. This is the difficult part of the practice because of your mental habits. You are so used to interpreting, calculating and analysing, which sweeps you away in more thinking rather than observing.

Mindfulness is about observation of interactions between thoughts, emotions, sensations and impulses, not controlling them. This also builds interoceptive awareness and helps your body in the process of multisensory integration.[13] This ability to observe is what helps your body to switch from threat mode to safety. Remaining an observer is hard. As is remaining curious and compassionate. But these attitudes are fundamental to the practice.

I went to see the grandfather of mindfulness himself, Jon Kabat-Zinn, about a year and a half into practising mindfulness at a packed-out conference hall in King's Cross. From his podium, he talked of the issues with the name 'mindfulness'. The connotations of the name were that it was all about thinking (i.e. mastering the dorsal thinking regions of the brain). This was a shame, he said, because it overlooked perhaps the most fundamental element of mindfulness: the spirit and feeling with which you practise it; the attitude of compassion and open-heartedness. Jon said that upon reflection, he'd much prefer that mindfulness was called 'heartfulness'.

As he said it, I felt myself having an 'aha' moment. My experience of mindfulness practice and training had been as much about befriending my experiences, however difficult they were, as it had been about gaining space from thoughts and mental filters. Compassion had been at the heart of my practice, albeit implicitly. An attitude of, *'Hey, this sucks, let's see how we can navigate this'*, rather than, *'WHAT ARE YOU DOING ABOUT THIS? DO IT BETTER!'* In the last chapter I described sitting beside yourself in solidarity for all the suffering you have experienced and how transformative that can be. This cultivation of compassionate solidarity with yourself is one of the lesser-known or communicated elements of mindfulness, but arguably one of the most powerful.

Traditional MBSR programmes have been shown to reduce anxiety, rumination and stress by increasing self-compassion.[14,15] Other studies show that mindfulness practice that *explicitly* cultivates self-compassion, can even be more effective in reducing anxiety and depression than mindfulness training alone.[16] Practising mindfulness with a compassionate attitude to yourself is necessary to regulate the ventral (emotional) brain regions so that the dorsal (thinking) regions don't go into overdrive (overthinking, rumination or worry). This is necessary to regulate difficult mood states and even physical symptoms.[17]

Brain imaging research shows that mindfulness practice engages areas of the brain that are involved in empathy and self-acceptance, such as the ACC and the insula.[18] These changes in the brain enhance emotional regulation and interoceptive awareness, reducing automatic threat-mode activation and aiding your brain in processing multisensory information.[19,20] Long term, as well as changing brain connectivity, mindfulness can alter the structure of the brain.[21,22] This reflects the power of kind-hearted observation of your experience in changing your brain and body. The physiological benefits of mindfulness have been well documented in the general population[23] and across specific conditions like IBS, IBD, mental fatigue, fibromyalgia, cancer and chronic pain.[24,25,26,27,28,29]

Keen to test the parameters of mindfulness after my own personally transformative experience with it, my master's thesis explored the benefits of a mindfulness-based cognitive therapy intervention for people with progressive multiple sclerosis (MS). MS is a condition where the immune system mistakenly attacks the protective covering of nerve fibres in the central nervous system, creating multiple neurological symptoms like pain, shaking, imbalance, continence issues, or more. Symptomatology varies widely across individuals, with some experiencing long remissions from any symptoms. The people in our study had a prognosis that guaranteed their trajectory was going to get more disabling. And yet, in this relatively short period of time, participants experienced improvements in pain, fatigue, anxiety and depression.[30]

'Don't tell me to do mindfulness!'

Mindfulness was suggested to me at a time that I was having cameras up my urethra (that's the small pee hole, resting just under your clitoris and yes it was as sensitive as it sounds), bladder biopsies, dyes pumped into my bladder and much more. None of this invasive and painful exploration was managing to explain why I still had the painful burning, and far-too-frequent need to urinate.

On one of the days I was lugging myself back and forth from the bed to the ensuite toilet in my dad's little cottage, my dad came into the room seeing my distress and asked, 'If you have nothing in your bladder, why don't you try *not* going to the toilet? See if you can just notice it.'

I explained, my voice strained and needling, that it felt like I would wet myself if I didn't get to the toilet. That what I was feeling was a sensation you only get when you are in imminent danger of losing bladder control. I simply could not stop attempting to empty my bladder.

His suggestion came around the time he also suggested I try mindfulness. I'll admit, both suggestions at first made me feel utterly misunderstood and alone in my suffering. Although the intention was to help, what I felt was being implied was that I was overreacting to the physical sensation I was feeling. That somehow it wasn't *really* as bad as I was making it out to be and that if only I tried harder, it would feel better. With this, the responsibility for feeling better fell on my over-burdened shoulders. Once again, it felt like I was being asked to do the impossible: to find a way to be OK with this intrusive physical sensation.

While mindfulness is absolutely one of the main reasons that I no longer have bladder issues after a long few years of struggling (and in the end I am eternally grateful for the suggestion and guidance), there are issues with the suggestion of doing mindfulness.

One of the key problems relates to the lack of clarity on what it actually is. Increasing awareness of the term 'mindfulness' results in misconceptions: that it is a practice of thought control or relaxation or imagery. In some spheres what is being described as 'mindfulness' is a diluted version that leaves a sour taste – a familiar sense that you are being tasked with sorting out 'problematic thinking'. When mindfulness is suggested as a quick self-directed fix it perpetuates this stigma.

It *is* hard to convey the full depths of mindfulness and with that, the benefits of it. That is why it used to be standard practice of many NHS services delivering MBSR to offer the opportunity to watch a documentary of mindfulness in action before patients decided whether to start an eight-week MBSR programme. The documentary was an episode, 'Healing From Within', of Bill Moyers's series called *Healing and the Mind*,[31] which followed one of Jon Kabat-Zinn's early mindfulness groups. Over the course of around ninety minutes, you witness the transformation of people dealing with severe physical suffering (pain from injuries, lifelong diagnoses, terminal conditions) from sceptical to open-hearted and engaged.

In one clip, Jon wipes a tear away from a group member's eye as she practises inhabiting her body non-judgementally, while holding a yoga pose. This was the documentary that made me feel hopeful after months of resigning myself to a shell of my former self.

Instead of suggesting something so abstract as 'trying mindfulness', sharing the documentary, and even (if possible) offering to watch it together and discuss, may garner more hope and sense of support.

Developing a different relationship with your thoughts

Rather than a magic fix that will rescue you from a moment of distress, practising mindfulness is just that: a practice. You can liken it to going to the gym to build muscle. Every time you train, you intentionally pick up weights and do 'reps' (repetitions). The equivalent in mindfulness practice is what I call a 'formal practice', intentionally doing a guided or unguided mindfulness meditation. Bringing your mind back every time it wanders is a 'rep'. The more you *gently* escort your mind back, the better your 'form'. Increased length of observing without getting tangled in thoughts is the equivalent to increased muscle endurance (e.g. holding weights/positions for longer).

There is no compelling data to suggest a minimum practice time required for benefit. As with most things, it is more about the consistency. And so, your formal mindfulness meditation practices may be five minutes or forty-five minutes. Whatever works with your life and your brain. If you have a brain that feels threatened and trapped at the prospect of ten minutes, there is no point aiming for forty-five minutes. You can also practise mindfulness by relating to your everyday experiences with mindful awareness. Perhaps brushing your teeth or enjoying the sunshine or spotting a swell of anger rise. Just by utilizing the principles and practices in this book, you are already increasing your day-to-day mindful awareness.

The power of mindfulness is cumulative. That means, a mindfulness meditation is not always going to be the thing you need to reach for when you are in the throes of symptoms or feeling very distressed. When clients of mine, new to mindfulness, experience severe endometriosis flares or feeling sick and dizzy because of migraine attacks, I'd not suggest they use mindfulness necessarily. Mindfulness involves turning towards a difficult experience, finding space alongside it. When everything in your body is in acute threat mode, grappling with a formal mindfulness practice can cause more pressure than it's worth at the time. Much like when I was struggling with going back and forth to the toilet. I had not yet built up the relationship with my mind, body and emotions for attempted mindful observation of my urinary urge to render any benefits – just a lot of frustration.

What I recommend in moments of extreme physical and/or emotional overwhelm, is prioritizing comfort. In Chapter 4, we looked at 'feeding your body positive experiences' to help you feel safe and soothed. In Chapter 5, we looked at the practice of savouring and how to lean into comfort. Both practices can be approached mindfully, but the practices themselves are not focussed on mindfully turning towards the discomfort.

As you start to practise mindfulness, it may feel difficult, sometimes impossible, to cultivate. You'll find that it comes more spontaneously, with more ease and less judgement as you continue practising. You'll find that even in the toughest moments, you are able to relate to your experience in a way that offers relief and calm. Rather than an acute fix, think of mindfulness like this: a practice that you gradually cultivate over time, so that when you need it, it holds you. Jon Kabat-Zinn uses a beautiful metaphor for this, of weaving your parachute every day, so that it holds you when you have to jump.

Earlier, I shared some of Sam's story. How she had found more relief and calm in letting her thoughts come and go, instead of trying to control them. The process of creating separation from your thoughts (and emotions) so that you can relate to them as transitory events, separate from you, is called 'cognitive defusion'. It is a core element of mindfulness practice, and of acceptance and commitment therapy. Brain imaging studies show that cognitive defusion reduces emotional intensity quickly, deactivating emotion-processing brain areas (e.g. amygdala, hippocampus, thalamus).[32]

Letting thoughts go*

If you can, use the audio guidance for this practice as this will be easier. The steps of the practice are detailed below.

1. Anchor yourself in your body. Feel your breath and the sensations of contact between you and the surface you are on. You can keep coming back to this physical sense as a tether when your mind wanders off. Notice what is comfortable and stabilizing about how you feel in this position. Perhaps the temperature is comfortable, or you feel a sense of support in the chair you are in.
2. Now pick something that you have been mildly worrying about. Don't pick anything too anxiety inducing for the purpose of the exercise.
3. Bring the concern to mind. Notice what thoughts arise. Be clear on your intention: you are not trying to figure anything out or analyse or fix. You are simply practising being with a mental event observationally with space and non-reactivity. How does it feel to observe?
4. What other feelings come with thoughts? Note any impulses arising.
5. Don't worry if you find it hard to remain an observer – it is hard. You are training your brain and body to keep regulated and calm rather than reactive.
6. When you come to open your eyes, note the following:

   - What happened to the thoughts when you let them be there but didn't try to engage with them?
   - What happened to the emotional intensity?
   - What felt counterintuitive? Why do you think that is?

---

* Download the audio guidance at www.healthpsychologist.co.uk/itsallinyourbody

Retraining worry habits

The previous exercise might be particularly hard if you worry often or if the thought you picked was a 'sticky' thought (my own term for them). 'Sticky' thoughts are the thoughts that are very hard to resist thinking about, dragging you into mental spirals as you try to work things out or think things better. This happens when you worry. Cognitive neuroscience has found that your brain can quickly make worry processes habitual because it feels like you are solving a problem[33,34] as the same brain regions are active (PFC and amygdala). However, problem-solving is clarifying and closed-ended, whilst worry is spiralling and open-ended. You therefore need to help your brain spot the difference. Use the flow chart in Figure 25 to guide you through the steps to do this. Table 10 contains alternative responses to worry for retraining your brain.

When it's time to go deeper

Sometimes your brain has developed mental habits like worry that will benefit from retraining as described. Other times, the repetitive nature of thoughts may cluster around themes that deserve deeper consideration. Earlier, I gave the example of the automatic thought 'my symptoms are going to get worse' being fed by a deeper belief system about not being safe. Self-critical thinking can be a mental habit, developed from deeper negative beliefs about self-worth. Beliefs develop automatically from your experience of the world. People who have had lots of medical trauma or health uncertainty understandably have beliefs that they are not safe, or that they will not be rescued when they need it. People who have been rejected or abandoned in times of immense vulnerability, may develop beliefs about being insignificant or unworthy. Others

Table 10: Worry types and related strategies

Type of worry	Description	Response options
Present worry within your control	Something that is happening and concerning you now that you have some influence over, e.g. not knowing what health appointments you have coming up. You can check your emails, phone and diary to get clarity and organize your schedule Remember, pinning down specifics of worry already reduces the mental load creating overwhelm	Swap worry with problem-solving: Specify the problem Generating solutions (ideally written down) Select one to try Plan in the steps to action solution or action right away Uncertainty of whether it will work may nag at you, but part of the worry habituation process is bearing with the feelings and seeing what happens.
Present worry outside of your control	Something playing out now, but you have no discernible influence over them, e.g. not knowing when you will be booked for a health appointment you need and not being able to expedite the booking	•**Letting thoughts go**: Use exercise on page 212. **Inhabit the present:** Engage with something intentionally in the present that can meaningfully tether your attention, e.g. focussing on a task like tidying or connecting with a loved one. Being able to come back to the present has a regulating effect on mind and body.[36,37] Having a specific tether (action, focal point) allows you to do this more easily.

Future or hypothetical worry	Something concerning that has not yet happened and may not happen, e.g. fearing that the appointment will be a waste of time	**• Positive distraction:** Allow your mind to be passively engaged to reduce emotional intensity, e.g. doing a puzzle or watching an engaging programme. Research shows that distraction does have a place in reducing anxiety and can physiologically reduce activation in the threat-processing part of the brain.[38] It can be particularly effective when you are having a high volume of thoughts that feel really important to figure out or very distressing to think about.[39] **• Imagery:** When you are worrying, you are having lots of 'verbal' thoughts that are conversational, generating more questions to be answered. Imagery helps switch your brain out of this mode. Imagine the best possible outcome, or even just a neutral outcome, to what you are worrying about. Picture it like a movie playing out and notice how that feels. Often this has an instantaneous recalibrating effect where the brain realizes that the negative outcome(s) it's been pouring over aren't a given. **• Permission to come back:** Sometimes it is hard to persuade that managerial part of you that it is not that big of a risk to stop thinking about the worry. Negotiate by agreeing an explicit time to come back to review the issue. Honour the time you choose to build trust with yourself. Make a point of reflecting on whether the worry still feels as big, present and threatening. If not, why not? What can you take from that?

who have relentlessly battled systems, advocated hard and still feel no further ahead may have beliefs about being powerless or the world being an uncaring, hostile place. You may appreciate that the beliefs arising from these experiences don't seem far-fetched. Working with them doesn't mean disproving them, it means understanding their scope and influence and working with them to mitigate the negative effects. Much of my clinical work is dedicated to unpicking belief systems that are too rigid, too overwhelming and sometimes wholly inaccurate. More on this in Chapter 8.

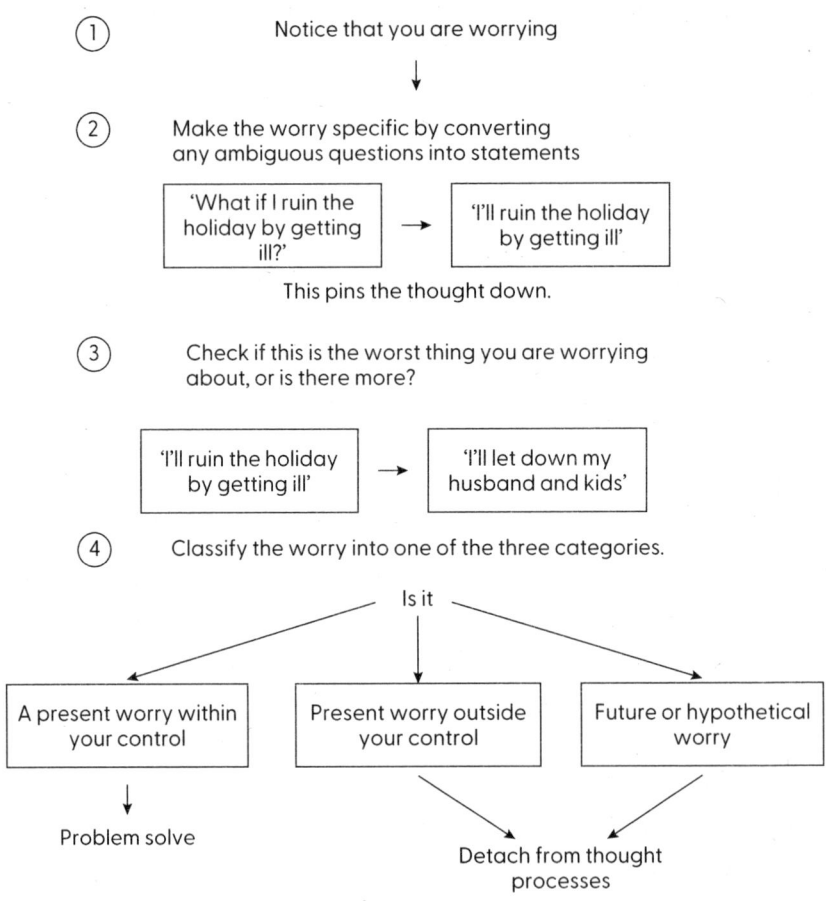

Figure 25: Sequence for retraining worry habits from Hirsch's Cognitive Process model[35]

Powers of placebo and nocebo

Your positive expectations about your health can influence your actual health outcomes. This is called the placebo effect. The opposite effect exists too. Negative expectations that medication won't work or that you'll have side effects can make these outcomes more likely.[40] It is estimated that as much as 80% of side effects are due to nocebo.[41] Both effects are widely demonstrated across research studies, with placebo effects being shown in the context of 'sham' surgeries as well as administration of placebo medications. Placebo and nocebo effects range from small to large and vary across conditions and symptomatology (e.g. pain, migraine, sleep, depression, fatigue, respiratory diseases and more). Different factors including context, gender and psychology make them more or less likely.[42]

Placebos create biological changes in your body that resemble the changes from the active drug you're expecting to receive. This led researchers to question, how much of the observed effects of active treatments are actually the result of the placebo effect? This is why all research trials require a placebo comparative condition.

How your body changes its physiology according to your expectations is complex and will differ across contexts and individuals. Men are more susceptible than women to the placebo effect especially when receiving information about the substance from a doctor. Whereas women are more likely to experience nocebo effects which are heavily informed by doctor–patient interactions.[43] These differences are likely due to the different healthcare experiences men can expect versus those women can expect. More on this in Chapter 7.

Placebo and nocebo can be another bittersweet discovery, because it puts emphasis on your own expectations. If you are trying a treatment and feel unsure or ambivalent about whether it will work, you may worry that you are preventing it from working. Here's why that doesn't have to concern you.

Although on one level, explicit thoughts about whether treatments will work do influence the placebo/nocebo effect, they are by no means the definitive factor. A big part of how the placebo and nocebo effect work is through associative learning processes in the brain that work on a more subconscious level to prime your body to respond.[44] The ritual of taking your medication each day as instructed can trigger associations in the brain that produce positive change. It's a bit like thinking you can't do an assignment. You have lots of thoughts and difficult feelings about it, but just by showing up, opening your laptop, getting out your stationery and pulling up the materials you need, your brain gets oiled up to respond as it has many times before to allow you to do the assignment. It starts to recognize it can do it because of the contextual cues that help it to process in that way – even if you are still having thoughts of *'I can't do this'*. These thoughts aren't all-powerful nullifiers.

You don't need to put extra pressure on how hopeful or negative your thoughts are about treatments. Studies show people can still experience the placebo effect for things like pain relief, fatigue and depression, when they are explicitly being told that they are receiving a placebo.[45] One fascinating qualitative study explored people's experience of taking a placebo.[46] One participant said:

'I wouldn't say I came with a bad attitude, but . . . I did not think that the placebo effect would work on me.'

Even for this participant, symptom severity scores of IBS fell dramatically, showing just how little the explicit thought processes can matter.

Extrapolating findings from this study and the broader research, here are some tips for maximizing the physiological benefits of the placebo effect and minimizing the negative side effects of the nocebo.

Table 11: Nocebo and placebo strategies

Maximizing placebo	Minimizing nocebo
Clarify with your health practitioner Find a trusted healthcare practitioner or allied healthcare practitioner that you can discuss your treatment with. Clarifying concerns, being heard and informed is fundamental to improving outcomes.	**Reframe side effect information** You can lower side effects by reframing side effect risk explicitly. E.g. a side effect with a 2% likelihood means that 98% are side-effect free. It may seem trivial, but research shows it reduces nocebo.[47]
Being proactive Associative learning processes in your brain that facilitate positive physiological changes can be activated by intentionally engaging with health actions. Create habits, routines and rituals that you consciously connect with the intention to improve your health. E.g. when taking medication, rather than gulping down with water, you might pair with enjoyable food (depending on medication) or a relaxed moment and have an enjoyable drink to follow up. When you do take the tablets consider the ways it is helping your body (even if you are cloudy on details).	**Remind yourself of nocebo** Just by knowing that the nocebo effect exists can reduce its likelihood or curtail nocebo side effects should they arise. More studies are needed to quantify the degree of impact this has.
Engage with positive feelings Motivation, hope and enthusiasm wax and wane, regardless of whether you have positive expectations about treatment procedures or health rituals. However, savouring and amplifying moments of feeling enthusiastic, curious or hopeful, can have a big impact on your biology resulting in positive health outcomes (page 190 – Chapter 5).	**Create a coping plan** Much like with the problem-solving approach explored previously, having engaged with potential avenues for dealing with side effects and what your options are, can reduce side effects and improve quality of life.[48]
Tackle underlying beliefs Your expectations of treatment are informed by deeper-level beliefs you hold. Beliefs like 'medications are toxic' or 'nothing works for me' can be rigidly held. Use Chapter 8 to explore strategies for introducing flexibility that may harness placebo and reduce nocebo.	

Imagining you are OK: the power of imagery

One of my clients, Yassim, had been in a terrible car accident resulting in full body burning pain. He felt this pain daily. It was clear that his pain was linked with the trauma of the car accident and his brain was perceiving that he was still in threat of being burnt alive. We did some trauma processing using EMDR. As part of this, we created a 'safe space', the visualization of a place that feels totally safe or comfortable and pleasant. For Yassim, this was being submerged in a water pool, which was the only time he didn't feel pain. We built this imagery and within minutes Yassim was telling me how pleasant and calm it felt. He could feel the water on his skin. When I asked him if he felt any pain, he reported none at all.

In a comprehensive meta-analysis, it was concluded that visualization practices physically improved pain, blood pressure, asthmatic symptoms of wheezing and muscle activation after surgery.[49] Just how powerful imagery is, almost has to be seen to be believed (irresistible pun). To illustrate, I return to the study I mentioned in the Introduction, that found that people in rehabilitation who rehearsed mental imagery of lifting heavy objects, without lifting anything, had increases of muscle strength of up to 136%. Mental imagery can positively affect multiple allostatic processes including inflammation, immune system function and heart rate.[50,51] When you mentally visualize a scene or series of images, you are activating neural pathways in the PFC, visual cortex and insula. Many of which are the same pathways that would be active if you were actually experiencing what you are imagining. The insula integrates emotional states with sensory information and converts these images into bodily sensations. The hypothalamus then alters the production of hormones, with a soothing effect on other psychobiological processes in the body.

As well as improving health experiences, imagery can have a

powerful impact on your motivation, confidence and ability to meet goals you set yourself.[52,53]

> **Creating a safe space**
>
> 1. Pick a place, real or imagined, that would make you feel safe, calm or at ease. Bring this place to mind in as much vivid detail in your mind's eye with your eyes closed. Note colours, textures and shapes that bring the image into clear view. What is the quality of the light? Where are you in the scene? How does your body feel? If you have aphantasia (where you are unable to visualize mentally) rather than closing your eyes, narratively describe it by writing.
> 2. Practise this imagery (in whatever way you can) over the course of three to five minutes. You can do longer if you like. Pay attention to how your body feels in this scene, how you feel and what it is like to inhabit this 'safe space'.
>
> This practice recalibrates your nervous system state, bringing it closer to balance, helping your body and brain feel safer.

Influencing your mental state

A pivotal part in my journey, was observing how my mental state was interacting with my physical and emotional states and feeling empowered to change that. I was fortunate that rather than shut down after my initial defensiveness, my dad gently encouraged me to explore mindfulness further. The change in my mental state was as much down to my dad's companionship of my explorations into mindfulness as it was the practice itself. He dutifully accompanied me in my early practice, setting the mats out, watching the documentary, buying me books and even in later years driving me to mindfulness retreats in the middle of the countryside. As I observed my thoughts, from a place of increasing regulation, I saw the errors my brain had been making. I wasn't as alone as I had assumed and even where people couldn't fully understand my experience, it didn't mean that they weren't trying to reach me. That was an immense comfort. Spending time with my thoughts changed my relationship with my body and myself, but it also helped me feel more connected. Shared human experience or a sense of common humanity is a recognized dimension of mindfulness that is fundamental to healing.[54] Neuroscience research shows that oxytocin (hormone involved in bonding) increases neural plasticity, which suggests that by practising mindfulness (or other learning activities) *collectively*, you can enhance your brain's ability to change.[55]

In this chapter, we've covered:

- The biological basis of thoughts, mental states and brainwave activity
- The relationship between your thoughts, attention and beliefs
- How to update common mental habits, including worry, rumination and self-criticism
- Myth-busting mindfulness and its place in health and illness
- How to start harnessing the power of placebo and imagery.

As you come to the end of this chapter, hopefully any sense of pressure you had to correct 'faulty' thinking has dissipated a little. Rather than taking on more things to control or drastically change, the invitation is for you to explore releasing some of that obligation. Doing so retrains your brain processing to be more regulating towards your regulatory systems.

Just as it was important for me to acknowledge how my dad's supportive encouragement impacted my mental state, it is important for you to consider your social world and how that impacts yours. Earlier we considered how your brainwave states can be influenced by your environment. Throughout this book, I've sought to counterbalance narratives of sole personal responsibility for healing with recognition of the interconnection between biology, psychology and social experiences. In the next chapter, we're going to explore this more centrally. Humans, after all, evolved to survive together, not in single silos.

CHAPTER 7

It's not all on you

My symptoms started just after I left university. Out of the blue and shocking at the time, in retrospect it makes sense. University was the first time I felt a sense of belonging and community. As an only child from a small, separated family, I had never felt the omnipotent sense of knowing that someone would always be around physically or emotionally. Until university, it was often the opposite – no one would be around.

Moving into halls and living with others who were also figuring out who they were, I felt a sense of cohesion. The vibrant nightlife, clubs and societies and the consistent presence of housemates. It was as glorious as it was messy. I was part of something, just by being *me* and being there.

This came to a pretty abrupt end when university was over. People moved back to their hometowns or to new exciting cities, while I remained, lost in my path and unknowingly grieving what I'd had: the safety of a collective experience. It was a big loss that part of me realized but failed to fully acknowledge, much less so see the link with my bladder issues. We aren't taught about the huge biological role our social environment and experiences have. How can something outside of us, as ethereal as a sense of connection, change the cellular activity in our body?

This chapter will share the fascinating, biology-altering power of your social experiences and your interconnection with the world around you. This will clarify why feeling alone, judged and solely responsible for your wellbeing, instigates a physiological threat response, and why a sense of belonging and strong social bonds can be so healing. We'll also explore how common socially threatening experiences interact with physical and mental health outcomes, including gender inequality, racism and ageism.

It can feel disempowering to acknowledge that something so vast, and so potentially out of your control, can have such a big impact. But don't worry, because I'll also address what you can do even when wider social experiences and societal issues are outside of your direct control. Rather than daunt you, this can excite you, opening your mind to the realms of opportunity to feel better in every sense of the word.

Social barometer

'Social safety' is the degree to which you feel safe from social threats like exclusion, rejection, hostility or neglect. Social safety has always been fundamental to the physical safety of humans, so much so that evolution favoured caring and sharing predispositions.[1] Your brain monitors your external world, combining that data, with what you are feeling (physically and emotionally) and thinking to determine social safety. This is a lot of data to process at any given, perhaps fast-moving, moment. Humans have evolved a 'social barometer' that allows fast calculations and communication between brain regions (e.g. amygdala, ACC) determining social safety and the regulatory systems and nervous system.[2] This allows the anticipation of social threat (like a conflict with a doctor or abandonment by a friend) to arouse activation in the immune system, which releases cytokines.[3] Cytokines are key messengers of the immune system, allowing it to deploy defensive action against pathogens. When they are released they can cause fatigue, headaches, body aches and brain fog. This explains why you can feel physically wiped out just by anticipating a bad time socially or why after an argument you can get a pulsing headache or nausea. When you repeatedly feel socially unsafe (e.g. lots of hostility, rejection or neglect) your immune system may remain activated or reactive, which can lead to increased long-term inflammation, autoimmunity and pain.[4,5]

To feel socially safe, your brain has to be able to register the presence of cues of safety. Cues of social safety can be verbal (e.g. warm tone), non-verbal (e.g. smile), environmental (e.g. soft lights, comfortable seating), relational (e.g. being accepted) or internal/interoceptive (e.g. slower breathing, warmth). You have magical little brain cells called 'mirror neurons', dedicated to helping you detect these safety cues. Your mirror neurons activate to help you infer what someone's intentions are or how they are feeling without the need for conscious thought. They are the reason you may automatically smile when someone smiles at you. Your mirror neurons alert you to the subtlest cues and even others' ANS arousal so that the slightest glance from someone can help you pick up on their mood and even feel a little of what they feel. Studies show that mirror neurons can synchronize your breathing, heart rate and pupil dilation with another person.[6] They can even mimic the physical pain of others.[7]

Genetics, personality, past experiences and neurodevelopmental differences impact your brain's ability to register safety cues and utilize mirror neurons. Both are enhanced by a sense of belonging. Belonging is the extent to which you feel personally accepted, included and supported by others in your social environment.[8] That social environment might be the company/setting you are in right now, or a broader environment. Interpersonal experiences and physical environmental factors like cleanliness, lighting or sounds can increase a sense of belonging and social safety.[9] Research shows that the features of your immediate physical environment can impact your healing and health trajectories. Patients who recovered in rooms with windows overlooking greenery were discharged faster, required less intense medications and had less post-operative complications than those recovering in rooms facing grey concrete.[10]

By now you may be getting the picture that when your brain perceives safety, your regulatory systems are better able to bring your body back to homeostasis (balance) for optimum healing and mental wellbeing. In those moments of practising mindfulness alongside my dad, or being soothed in my sorrow by my partner, although I was physically and mentally struggling, I was being nourished by multiple cues of social safety and a high sense of belonging. In the moment it didn't magic my pain away – it didn't even feel much like belonging – but it did allow my body and I to find our way back to some sense of balance.

Socially threatened

'Social threats' may be:

- **Relational**: social exclusion, rejection, hostility or neglect, etc.
- **Financial**: financial insecurity, poverty
- **Systemic**: unjust or punitive legal, healthcare, educational, political systems
- **Environmental**: poor housing, noise pollution, pollution, etc.

Social threats can exist with varying proximity to you across different rungs of social spheres that exist around you (in your peer/family group, broader community, workplace, city, country or the world). For example, climate change poses a world threat, but it may affect you more proximately if you have wildfires in your country or individually if your house was burnt down by them. The more proximate the threat feels to you, the greater the disruption to your sense of safety, generally. Some broader social threats with less direct individual proximity may still elicit a high degree of threat, such as war. Social threats can affect your core safety needs as identified in the power threat meaning framework: basic needs, safe relationships/attachment, control, fairness, personal sense of value and meaning.[11]

Financial insecurity is one of the greatest threats to your sense of social safety because it threatens all core safety needs, including the basics (e.g. food, shelter, healthcare). Just the *prospect* of not being able to cover your basic needs, is enough to dysregulate the neuroendocrine, metabolic, cardiovascular and immune systems. Financial strain can therefore make you more susceptible to heart-related issues, including heart attacks, respiratory infections and autoimmune diseases.[12]

How you are treated or anticipate being treated by systems and communities you access (e.g. education, local government, workplace) will shape your perception of safety. Public policy, messaging and behaviour of others in these settings will create 'social safety schemas'.[13] These are brain-made templates to anticipate social threats, with the power to determine how you interpret social experiences (e.g. whether a smile is a smile or a smirk). Social safety schema can also initiate a full range of biological interactions, including activation of the SNS and HPA axis, affecting your behaviour and physical and mental health.

Healthcare system experiences can be extremely threatening. When you are treated like a number rather than an individual, you can lose trust that your welfare and safety is being prioritized.[14] Mistrust is understandably exacerbated by inattentive, dismissive or hostile bedside manners. Areas of your brain that process trust (or mistrust) are areas of the brain that are involved in risk, positive anticipation, social hostility and pain.[15] If you have experienced lots of medical negligence, trauma or hostility in the healthcare system, your brain calculates high risk, high hostility and high physical pain (or risk thereof) with little reward, making it hard for you to believe that you will be looked after. This calculation transmits to your nervous system telling it you need to be on guard. As it activates, the release of hormones and neurotransmitters can make you physically feel even more vulnerable as your heart races, breath quickens and thoughts whir. Many of my clients have experienced medical trauma. Sometimes just having to call for a routine appointment can elicit fear, procrastination, nausea and worry. Social threats like these have also been shown to increase physical pain. As explored in Chapter 2, brain areas that process social experiences also process pain and emotion.[16]

Unfortunately, Western, individualistic societies that prize achievement and capitalistic pursuits (like the accumulation of wealth) tend to make those more vulnerable or requiring of support, feel socially excluded or rejected. The implicit shared assumption of societies like these is that if you can't 'contribute' as much (monetarily) and you require more support, you are personally defective. These messages are transmitted in the media with headlines like 'benefit scroungers', in public policy that treats recipients of social support with suspicion and in the absence of equality of access to things like public transport.[17] In London, for example, wheelchair users cannot guarantee that they can exit from the station they wish to because of insufficient and unreliable lift access. In more recent years, with increasingly polarizing political and social commentary, we even see prominent politicians and entertainers openly mocking disability, with no real repercussions.

These social threats permeate through the various social spheres, so that even if you are never explicitly mocked or criticized for your mental health or physical illness, you may feel at risk of it. Humans are distinctly porous to social threat messaging. When symptoms were making it hard to concentrate at work and I couldn't be as diligent as usual, I felt like I was failing. I dreaded going into the office because I felt ashamed. These feelings were heavily influenced by societal conditioning. As are the sentiments of being a 'burden' or 'drain', when you're ill or dealing with mood difficulties. You've been conditioned to think these things, but they are by no means true. Because if you hold that assumption up to the light, you'll see that what it is explicitly saying is 'if you experience any vulnerability, you are weak and failing'. And if that is true, then it is acceptable to abandon people when they are at their most depleted. Not only is this incredibly callous and cruel, but it is also fundamentally untrue. All humans, whether you like to admit it or not, are vulnerable. It's just a case of whether their circumstances have shown them that or not.

Your subconscious defences

In Chapter 5, we explored the defences your brain and body have for highly distressing emotions. In evolutionary terms, social threats posed significant danger to human survival, so our brains and bodies still take such threats very seriously. In modern society, there are more social threats than ever. You are in contact with more people via the internet, transport advances and city design. Social media, forums and websites tell you the opinions of hundreds of thousands of people on any given day, which makes social approval even more of a currency. You have more metrics for determining whether you are acceptable or included than ever before (e.g. likes, views). Your brain processes more markers of social threat than it receives of social safeness.[18,19]

Neuroscience research shows that when you feel personally inadequate, often in relation to social exclusion or rejection, the brain tries to protect you. It can do this through a process called 'cognitive deconstruction', whereby you disconnect from your emotions, your sense of self and even higher order thinking.[20] Cognitive deconstruction is characterized by emotional numbing, lethargy, avoidance and internally focussed thoughts. This is what I experienced those times where I was monosyllabic, unwilling and unable to engage, trapped with self-hating thoughts. Cognitive deconstruction has short-term benefits in numbing the pain of being socially excluded or feeling personally defective. Long term it is associated with significant mental health difficulties.

Another intuitive protection against social threats is to withdraw. Although understandable, it precludes you from the hugely protective and restorative benefits of social connection.[21] Access to safe social connection has the power to reduce risk of serious illness and increase healthy life years because of its ability to restore bodily homeostasis and buffer against the psychobiological effects of stress.[22,23] The automatic intuition to withdraw therefore withholds nourishment and increases depletion. We'll explore counterbalancing options later.

The final defence is one that we considered back in the Introduction. That is the polarized perceptions your brain creates to determine your role in your suffering. It may either determine that you have no influence at all and that you are powerless in the face of cruel societal structures that will keep you stuck no matter what. Or that your suffering is your personal responsibility to mend. Both can be disempowering, inhibiting healing and connection.

Reclaiming control without overburdening yourself

Brains 'like' to buy into self-defective narratives (believe it or not) telling you that *you* are the problem because this creates potential for control and therefore safety. Self-help books tend to focus solely on what *you* need to do to improve things, which can feel empowering. However, failure to recognize the role of social context can fuel self-stigmatizing senses of over-responsibility for healing and improvement. This can imply the corrosive idea that 'if you are still suffering, you're not trying hard enough. You. Are. The. Problem.' The personal responsibility rhetoric sees workers that are working way beyond reasonable hours thrown a 'wellbeing day' to help them take further responsibility for their stress, while the organization fails to address workload issues. It sees people who are financially destitute blamed for their illnesses by media tabloids without acknowledgement of how hard it is to preserve health when time is sparse, money is tight, and stress is at an all-time high.

'You are the problem' is a corrosive idea that is very hard to shift. For this reason, you need to be aware of, and receive acknowledgement for, how your social experiences and wider society impacts you. The truth is that it can never be all on you.

Humans are interdependent beings, and we have always relied on the support of others to survive and thrive. We are still biologically predisposed to require social safety for our health and wellbeing.

You deserve social structures that support you and to feel socially connected. The following sections aim to provide acknowledgement of *some* of the societal experiences that affect some groups. Please note, there are many more groups affected by social stigmatization and hardship that are not included here. Those of you marginalized for things I've not captured (your sexuality, transness, religion, weight, class, appearance), your experiences matter and they deserve acknowledgement. I've chosen to write about the ones I know best, and are not a reflection of the ones I deem to be most deserving of acknowledgement. I hope that consideration of these examples can go some way to help process and understand your own societal injuries.

Girl, you're crazy!

If you are a woman dealing with physical health issues, unfortunately, it is more likely than not, that you have been told your physical symptoms are the result of your mental health. The attribution of women's health ailments to psychological causes has been happening for centuries. Ancient Greek physicians like

Hippocrates believed that a 'wandering womb' would roam the body dissatisfied until impregnated. This wandering was to blame for symptoms ranging from headaches to infertility. The cure for a wandering womb was pregnancy.

Unfortunately, attitudes haven't evolved as much as you might hope. People with severe endometriosis and adenomyosis (conditions that can cause intense pain and internal bleeding) are not uncommonly told to *get pregnant*. Please be aware, there is no medical evidence for this helping either condition and there can be difficulties in getting pregnant, so this is particularly cruel and misguided advice.

In the Victorian era, physicians like Sigmund Freud created a handy catch-all for women's health complaints: 'hysteria'. Physical health issues of women were presumed to be due to female-specific neurosis and many were prescribed the 'rest cure', which was to lie in bed and limit movement. Unsurprisingly this led to further mental and physical deterioration, which generally was attributed to the woman's weak-mindedness.

Despite medical advances, the sense that women cannot be trusted to accurately report the extent of their own physical suffering continues. In a UK government survey, 84% of women reported having not been listened to by healthcare professionals.[24] A prior report investigating similar issues with medical misogyny, stated that in the NHS there was a 'culture of dismissive and arrogant attitudes that only serve to intimidate and confuse.'[25] This bias and treatment of women physically impacts health and psychologically breeds fear and mistrust. Women wait longer in emergency departments for pain meds than men when reporting abdominal pain, they are less like to be prescribed pain medication compared to men and they are more likely than men to have symptoms of a heart attack dismissed as a panic attack, anxiety or indigestion.[26,27,28] If you can't trust that you will be taken seriously and given the medical support you require when the control is out of your hands, it is incredibly hard for your brain and body not to stay vigilant. This constitutes a huge threat, so your body responds by trying to remain alert to mitigate it. Being told that what you are experiencing isn't real can create disruption to your interoceptive awareness and multisensory integration. Your brain therefore becomes more likely to alert you to neutral bodily signals as though they are threats,[29,30] thereby increasing physical discomfort and health issues.

So, 'girl', you're not crazy. You are not being listened to and that can make you feel crazy. Let this information marinade into your subconscious, so that when you doubt yourself or feel alone in your suffering, there is a little seed inside that remembers you can trust yourself and there are women worldwide experiencing this and committed to changing your plight.

Man, you got it bad too!

While men have the privilege of being more likely to be taken seriously by a doctor, what they don't have so much (societally) is the permission to feel and explore negative emotions. Gendered stereotypes see women as the feelers and men as the doers. Men are expected to be stoic, 'strong' and are glorified for exerting dominance, self-promotion and assertiveness. These are perceived as positive signs of confidence and leadership in men, who are then more likely to get promoted for it, when compared to women for whom these traits are seen as arrogant and selfish.[31] While again there is an inherent privilege in this, there is also a dark downside for men.

When feeling or displaying vulnerable emotions is socially unsafe, it feeds internalized shame and prevents the acknowledgement of feelings. Some colleagues and I compared interviews of men versus women with bladder pain syndrome. I was astounded by the stark contrast in how genders considered the impact on emotional wellbeing. While women were quick to talk about the emotional toll, in the men's interviews it wasn't mentioned until a specific question prompted the consideration, to which the response was along the lines of, 'Huh, hadn't really thought much about that'.[32]

When masculine stereotypes are internalized (knowingly or not), men will tend to push away or ignore vulnerable feelings and emotional openness with others.[33] This may account for why only 36% of referrals for free therapy on the NHS were for men[34] and why once in therapy, men are more likely to discontinue prematurely.[35] I have seen first-hand how these societal messages of being weak, or undeserving of emotional support, cause men in therapy to wrestle with their conscience about being in therapy. These messages create internalized beliefs that prevent engagement in therapy, which can play out in various ways: questioning the use of specific words or phrases in therapy discussions, intellectualizing or storytelling, doubting the adequacy of the therapist and avoiding home practices. If these beliefs aren't sufficiently worked with, it can add to feelings of shame and intensify emotional suppression.[36]

Shame and suppression affect biological processes which shape health/illness. Men generally have shorter life expectancies than women and some of this is explicable by the fact that men engage in more risk-taking behaviour, like the pursuit of high adrenaline sports or fast driving, and they tend to drink more alcohol and smoke more.[37] These pursuits may well be driven in part by the expectation to suppress feelings and vulnerabilities. Indeed, research shows that men have fewer close friendships that entail open, explorative conversation, than women.[38]

Emotional suppression and internalized shame may also go some way to explain why suicide is the leading cause of death for men aged 50 and under in the UK.[39] Normalization of emotional suppression wears the body down over time. Suppression is linked to increased amygdala activation and ANS reactivity, which perpetuates emotional overwhelm. This repeated pattern over time reduces the PFC's ability to regulate emotions and utilize helpful coping strategies. This increases hopelessness, making it seem like there are limited options and from this place suicide can quickly feel like the only option.

If you are a man reading this and you find it hard or awkward to be emotionally open with many others, you may find yourself often doing things to drown out emotional discomfort like being glued to your devices, constantly trying to think your way out of problems and perhaps drinking more than you'd like or excessively exercising. The second half of this chapter will give you alternative options, and the next chapter will help you explore in more depth.

Societal expectations of gender can affect everyone to some degree. Whether you are a woman perceived as overly anxious. Or a man fearing judgement of being weak for having vulnerability. Or you are trans or non-binary, negotiating your pronouns and uncertain of what hostility you might face. It is important to understand your brain and body process quicker than you consciously think. So adept are they to determining social threats, that certain situations or contexts may make you feel more self-conscious, anxious or conspicuous without you necessarily realizing why (e.g. woman going into GP surgery, man going to therapy, transperson going to a conservative event).

'Where are you *from* from?' effects

In most of the Western world, forms capturing demographic information, have White Caucasian as the default check box. Yet the majority of the world's population is not White Caucasian. Colonial rule and exploitative historical events have meant that White people find themselves top of racial social hierarchies.[40] Consequently, in countries like the UK, USA and much of Europe, non-White people from diverse racial or ethnic backgrounds are often grouped under the umbrella term 'ethnic minority'. A term that can be considered othering of non-White races as it oversimplifies a multitude of racial identities, creating a universal 'minority' status for people who are in fact not the global 'minority' but the majority.

Othering can take various forms, some subtle through to violent attacks. Researchers have categorized racial discrimination into three types:[41]

- **Hostility:** open aggressive or demeaning behaviour towards someone based on their race like racial slurs, threats or violence
- **Aversive hostility:** passive-aggressive or systemic exclusion because of race, often characterized by othering microaggressions (e.g. 'Where are you *from* from?')
- **Avoidance:** passive rejection characterized by lack of interaction or engagement rather than hostility (e.g. lack of inclusion in group discussions in contrast to active inclusion of others).

Discrimination can happen at an individual level, within institutions (like the healthcare system) or culturally (i.e. the norm in your city or country).

As someone with a visually ambiguous heritage, frequently called a variety of racial slurs in school, I've always felt that racism is lurking underneath the niceties. I grew up with stories from my dark-skinned, Indian mum of her time in a majority White, middle-class grammar school after moving from India as a young child. I remember feeling horrified as she told me stories of how she would be punished for the racist behaviour of her peers – reprimanded for 'telling tales' or misunderstanding. In therapy, I've since heard similar stories, with many of my female Black clients labelled 'aggressive' when advocating for themselves. These are examples of hostility followed by aversive hostility.

Being discriminated against is a threatening experience. To have that discrimination implicitly approved of or accepted by others adds significantly to the social threat. Discriminatory experiences prime your body for defence (threat mode), with studies linking discrimination with increased allostatic load.[42] Other studies show that experiences of racism consequently increase the likelihood of having poorer physical health, including asthma, diabetes, arthritis and weight gain.[43]

Discrimination affects health in other ways too. Institutional racism puts ethnic minorities (global majorities) at risk of health complications and even increased death rates. A shocking study showed that Black women in the UK were five times more likely to die in childbirth than their White counterparts and Asian women were twice as likely.[44] This study has since been reviewed alongside others like it, highlighting shocking racial health disparities, in a paper published in *The British Medical Journal* warning against ignoring the role of racism and unconscious bias that contribute to these findings.[45]

Racism is senseless and unjust, making it particularly hard to process, whilst eroding your sense of empowerment and agency. We'll explore ways of dealing with these very real challenges, but in the meantime acknowledging how problematic social infrastructures can make you feel less than you are, how they can chip away at your worth along with your safety, is integral for starting to feel safe as you are. In the words of Maya Angelou, 'You may not control all the events that happen to you, but you can decide not to be reduced by them.' You are not the problem – the system is.

'I'm too old to change': Old dogs can learn new tricks

'Is it too late to get better?' I am often asked this by clients in their *twenties* and *thirties*. When you've experienced physical and/or emotional disruption for so long it can feel like you are 'too far gone'. Aside from the fear and misalignment with your body, part of the reason this may feel so persuasive is due to the narratives you have been fed about aging.

Views of aging and the elderly differ across cultures. Respect for elders is pronounced in non-Western cultures, including Eastern, African, Indigenous and Middle East cultures. The wisdom afforded from the life experiences of the elderly and the heritage and traditions they uphold, and of which they are the custodians, is cherished amongst these cultures.

In the West, where individualism and independence are glorified, aging is viewed negatively with a high emphasis on preventing it.[46] These attitudes can shape how you feel about yourself, making you feel less acceptable as you grow older. Turning 40 can mean different things to different people. It can mean, 'Oh my gosh, I'm hurtling into another decade towards being old and feeble', or it can mean, 'What a privilege, I've accrued so much more knowledge and know myself better'.

The connotations you have of aging shape your behaviour that impacts your health. If 'old' immediately comes with connotations of being less valuable – a burden, perhaps – decrepit, weak, vulnerable, then aging may be accompanied by fear. You are more likely to back away from physical activity for fear of falls and less likely to try and find alternatives that feel safe, as you feel doomed to your destiny of slow decay. In contrast, if you associate 'old' with wisdom, with growth and an increased knowing of yourself and your fellow humans, then you may feel more able to trust what you can do physically and mentally and be more inclined to do it.

My grandmother is my inspiration for this. At the tender age of 80-something, I found her frantically racing up and down the stairs looking for something. She'd already done her stint in the garden (her treadmill wasn't scheduled for today), and she'd been out to play bridge (third time that week). I asked her what she was doing, and she said that she must urgently sell some stocks as China had done something and the market was about to crash (it flew over my head, but that was the gist). As I watched her find her passwords for her stock accounts, breathing a sigh of relief upon selling her stocks, my amusement was surpassed by my awe at her tenacity. A few days later, the Chinese stock market crash was all over the news. Grandma is the antithesis of the idea that aging means you resign your mind and body to doing the bare minimum. She doesn't push her body beyond its capability, but she knows it well and she works with it expertly.

Neuroplasticity and bioplasticity are the brain and body's ability to adapt through the forming or strengthening of neural connections based on new experiences and learning.

Neuroscience research confirms that neuroplasticity continues into old age.[47] The rate and efficiency of forming or strengthening synaptic connections may decline, but you have lots of options at your disposal to preserve and enhance it. Lots of the research exploring neuroplasticity and old age combines it with the concept of bioplasticity as it explores the benefits specifically of exercise on neuroplasticity.

Both prior to old age and in old age, engaging in regular exercise (pitched to your capacity) preserves your brain's ability to change and update.[48,49] Specifically, a review of brain imaging studies on the effects of exercising in the brains of elderly people found that exercise induces changes in the hippocampus (important for memory and emotion regulation) and the cerebellum (coordination of balance, cognition and emotion).[50]

When it comes to these benefits, not all exercise is made equal. There is a difference between treadmill walking and dancing that has nothing to do with the degree of heart rate elevation or respiration. It has to do with how much it gives your brain a workout. Dancing is more demanding of your brain and cognitive processes, compared to treadmill walking which doesn't really demand much. Researchers took brain scans of participants who ranged between 63 and 79 years old, who did the same frequency and duration of exercise but differed in terms of how much 'cognitive load' it demanded. Over the course of four months, only those in the high cognitive load exercise group saw improvements in their cognitive function (better memory, reasoning, focus, etc.) denoted by increased connectivity in brain regions involved in these higher order thinking processes.[51] The brain imaging also showed decreased activation in two brain regions called the middle occipital gyrus and postcentral gyrus, suggesting that they were able to filter out visual distractions and feel less disruption from physical sensations.

The old saying 'use it or lose it' is misguiding, implying that if you don't consistently work your brain and body in particular ways, you'll be precluded from doing so later. Tell that to Grandma Moses, an American folk artist who took up painting after arthritis made it hard for her to embroider, gaining worldwide acclaim. Or Fauja Singh, who started running marathons at 89 years old! Or Nola Ochs who went back to university, aged 90, completing her degree at 95 and master's at 98. What these stories and this research shows, is that you don't lose 'it' per se. Whether that be cognitive ability or the ability to condition your body. A more hopeful and accurate phrase would be 'challenge fuels change at any age'. The more you challenge, the more you can change.

'What is wrong with you?' Neurodivergence

Neurodivergence is an umbrella term to describe people whose brains, cognitive processing and behaviours differ from typical neurological functioning and societal norms. Neurodivergence is a natural variation in brain function across humans rather than a condition to be cured. There are different types of neurodivergence, including attention deficit hyperactivity disorder (ADHD), autism, dyslexia, dyspraxia and Tourette's syndrome, each with different 'symptoms' or characteristics. I'll specifically consider ADHD and autism, but some of the problems faced and consequent social experiences often apply to the other neurodivergent conditions.

Table 12 gives a summary of symptoms seen in ADHD and autism.

Many of my neurodivergent clients share the experience of having been told explicitly and implicitly that there is something

Table 12: Summary of ADHD and autism	
Neurodivergent conditions	**Summary & characteristics**
Attention Deficit Hyperactivity Disorder (ADHD)	Broadly characterized by impulsivity, hyperactivity, and/or inattention. Symptoms may include losing focus mid-task, aversion to tasks that require sustained efforts causing avoidance, difficulties with distraction and memory, restlessness, making in-the-moment decisions without thinking it through, interrupting and difficulty waiting. Lots of these symptoms are experiences everyone has, but the degree and impact are much more severe for those with ADHD.
Autism Spectrum Disorder	Marked by differences in communication, social interaction, and sensory processing. Symptoms may include difficulties with social interactions such as finding eye contact uncomfortable, difficulty interpreting nonverbal communication or cues, or tending to be over literal or direct. There may be the tendency to have a strong attachment to routines with difficulty handling unexpected changes and with this there may be repetitive behaviour and intense focussed interests. Difference in sensory processing can mean that people with autism experience certain sensory experiences more intensely, such as lights, sounds and noises, or they seek strong sensory experiences like pressure.

wrong with them. School routines, adult expectations, societal niceties that their brains (particularly in childhood) could not easily understand or conform to, resulting in them being labelled 'naughty' or 'different'. These stigmas often follow people into their adult lives with an internalized pressure to conform to neurotypical norms that don't work for their brains and bodies, negatively impacting self-esteem. For those with neurodivergence who do manage to conform as expected ('masking' is the name for this process), it can cause significant mental and physical strain, which contributes to allostatic load,[52] emotional dysregulation and reduced capacity for influencing cognitive processes.[53]

These impacts on mental health and psychological processing interact with physical health. High emotional reactivity (or sensitivity) can change functioning of regulatory systems and the ANS tends to be more reactive in those with neurodivergence.[54] As you'll be familiar with by now, increased ANS activity changes biological processes that contribute to varied health problems like gut issues, chronic pain and changed immunity.

Neurodivergent cognitive processing can also impact physical health indirectly. Cognitive processing in neurodivergence can make all-or-nothing thinking (page 128) more likely.[55] All-or-nothing thinking lends itself to all-or-nothing behaviour that directly affects health: restrictive diets or rigid eating habits, over-exercising or avoidance of exercise and perfectionist tendencies towards health micromanagement. Changed cognitive and nervous system processing can dial up or dial down sensory signals, changing interoceptive awareness and multisensory integration (page 107). This can mean a heightened awareness and anxiety of physical symptoms and/or a lack of awareness, meaning basic bodily cues like hunger or thirst are missed.[56,57] As previously explored, disruptions to interoceptive awareness can impact homeostatic bodily balance and nervous system processing, contributing to physical symptoms and potentially cumulating allostatic load. For these reasons (and more not discussed here) there is a significant overlap between those with neurodivergence and physical health conditions.[58]

Increasing awareness of neurodivergence and the impact of the pandemic on those with neurodivergence has meant that more people are receiving diagnoses of ADHD and autism as an adult. The importance of getting a diagnosis in neurodivergence goes beyond the management options it opens. Diagnosis can diffuse self-stigma in a way nothing else will. Patients of mine who have received a diagnosis whilst working with me have had eureka moments, transforming their relationship with themselves. I had one client tell me, 'I make so much more sense to myself now! My brain just works differently.'

I love working with clients with ADHD and autism because they have so much insight into how their brain is working and can share hugely revelatory observations of their own cognitive processing. Because of this, I have gained some of my deepest insights into my work. The ability to lean into the biology of neurodivergence can create freedom and alleviate pressure. Therein lies a beautiful relationship with your mind and body.

We've considered how the brain and body process cues of social safety or threat subconsciously and automatically and how social experiences contribute to that. What has resonated with you, personally? What social messaging has affected your sense of safety or threat?

Maximizing social safety and mitigating social threats in so far as this is possible, is fundamental for restoring bodily balance. This is what the next section will explore.

How to feel socially safe

We've explored how you have an internal social barometer that allows your brain to quickly process information about you, your social interactions and environment.

The following practices will focus on working with your external world to update your social barometer and increase your sense of social safeness. We'll first consider navigating potentially hostile or excluding social experiences and then we'll go on to consider ways that will help you to build social safety through increasing social connectedness.

Advocating for yourself

It can be hard to voice your needs at the best of times – even more so when you are vulnerable or depleted. Many of my clients have felt voiceless and choiceless in their suffering. Clients with chronic fatigue, chronic pain or recovering from surgery have told me how they walked for longer than they should or went to work sooner than they were ready to because they felt guilty and unable to advocate for their own needs. When doctors have said abhorrent things like 'your weight is causing this' or 'there's no such thing as [insert health issue]', they've been rendered speechless. Many never make official complaints later for reasons they don't fully understand themselves.

We discussed gendered norms and how they contribute to health experiences. It is very common for women to have learnt to self-subjugate (put yourself last) as this is what society tells them they should do to be 'good'. This is learnt from a young age. It does not just apply to women. If growing up, regardless of gender, you were relied upon to be the sensible one, or the fixer, it is also likely that you learnt to put your own needs to one side. When self-subjugation is the norm, acting assertively can feel impossible. More than that, it can feel like a *bad* thing. That you'd be doing something wrong or mean. So, let's correct that notion by clarifying what assertiveness is.

Assertiveness is a way of communicating your thoughts, feelings, preferences or needs while being aware and respectful of others' thoughts, feelings, preferences and needs. Assertiveness is often confused with aggressive communication, which prioritizes oneself with no regard for others. You should think of assertiveness as a means of equalizing the balance between you and another, not tipping it completely in your favour. Table 13

Table 13: Spectrum of assertiveness

	Passive	Passive-aggressive	Assertive	Aggressive
	Avoiding expressing or advocating for your own needs.	Indirectly expressing negative feelings or needs often through sarcasm or apparent jokes.	Expressing yourself openly, honestly and respectfully, whilst being mindful of others. Assertiveness is cooperative and flexible within specified boundaries.	Expressing thoughts and preferences in a way that violates or disregards the rights of others often in a hostile, dismissive or domineering manner.
Saying no to a request when you are unwell	Um... OK... I can try.	Well, I am sick, but I suppose you can't do it without me.	I'm sorry, I'm not feeling well and need to rest, so I can't help right now. Can we revisit another time?	Why would you even ask me that when I'm sick? You're selfish!
Dealing with criticism from someone telling you that you always cancel last minute	I'm sorry, I'll try not to cancel any more.	It's not like I'm having a great time!	I understand it is frustrating that I have to cancel. I don't take it lightly, but I am unwell and have to look after myself. I'm sorry. Can you understand?	Seriously? If you can't understand that I've been sick, why the hell should I explain myself to you?
Asking for adaptations	I'll eat beforehand, don't worry about me. Looking forward to it.	Another night where I get to nibble on lettuce – guess I'll save money!	The restaurant looks lovely, but I've checked the menu and there aren't any options I can eat. Would you mind if we choose somewhere else? I can come up with options?	That's crap for me. Can you choose somewhere else that I might actually enjoy?

illustrates the difference between assertive, aggressive and passive communication.

In situations where your needs are not being considered or are being violated, you need to be able to advocate for yourself assertively. This includes making sure you receive the diagnostic procedures you require to get clarity on your health or having a loved one help you practically when you are incapacitated. The benefits of assertiveness go beyond receiving the help you ask for. Assertive communication can improve your mood and relationships, while also reducing anxiety.[59] In contrast, passive communication often breeds emotional suppression. In a study conducted by my colleague at King's College London, across interviews with patients with IBS, concerns about being approved of by others resulted in the bottling-up of emotions.[60] This is a pattern I recognize a lot in my clients regardless of specific diagnoses. Over time, bottling-up really stacks up, leaving your body to pay the price (Chapter 5).

The foundations of assertiveness

Saying no

No is a complete sentence, as my dad's friend used to say when I started replying to his questions with 'no because...'. You may often feel the need to elaborate and justify yourself to ensure that you are understood and the other person does not think badly of you. Although there may be a level of explanation required in the spirit of transparent, assertive communication, come back to this mantra: 'No is a complete sentence.' Below are some example situations where it may feel rude not to elaborate or white-lie even, but where it can increase your sense of self-acceptance and agency to simply say no.

- **Someone offers you food you cannot/do not want to eat**
  Them: Would you like one of these, they're really good!
  You: That's very kind, but no thank you.

You may feel the need to elaborate, likely in a self-deprecating way: 'Oh, I've eaten far too much already!' or a roll of the eyes 'I'm *trying* to be good.' Don't do it. You have every right to say you don't want something that you are offered. There is simply no need to apologize.

- **Someone asks you to do some extra work that is technically outside your remit**
  Them: Would you be able to fill out that form in time for the meeting on Friday?
  You: I don't usually work on those forms. It would be xxx or yourself. Do you need some support?

Here it can feel uncomfortable because you are saying no to a request for help. Just because you technically *could* help or have the capacity, doesn't mean you should always give it. It has a snowball effect that buries you in an avalanche, so the earlier you practise saying no to the things that are not within your remit, the more capacity you can preserve.

- **A doctor offers you a treatment option you don't feel comfortable with**
  Doctor: You could get started with this straight away. I can fill out the prescription now.
  You: I don't feel comfortable with that treatment because [your reasoning]. I had hoped for [your expectation]. Would it be possible to explore that?

Here you *are* explaining your reasoning which is important in the context. If the doctor knows your concerns, they are better able to work with you on finding a solution. You are also specifying your preferred outcome, which further helps this.

Asking for what you want

It can feel vulnerable to ask explicitly for what you want. In romantic relationships, it can feel embarrassing to be sexually open and directive. With family, it can feel scary to share your feelings if they've been dismissed before. Sometimes you can assume that what you want and need is obvious to others – particularly when they are close to you. It can feel upsetting when they don't automatically know, and your brain can infer that they don't know you or care that much. Often this is far from the truth. Their own emotional discomfort at your suffering can mean they are prohibited by their own brains to meet you where you are.

Long-standing relational patterns that mishandle your vulnerability (e.g. silence or jokes) don't have to be on repeat.

To change dynamics you have to find the words to say what is not working for you and what would work better. Your brain may already be saying, *'But what if they don't listen? I'll feel worse.'* This is a possibility, but often just expressing your preference is a relief. We'll talk a bit about working with the discomfort of not being met in your requests in a moment.

- **You feel unwell and unable to make dinner as planned with your other half**
  You: I know I said I'd cook, but I don't feel good at all. Are you able to cook tonight or grab us something easy from the shop?
  Them: I don't know what I'd make. Do you want a pizza?
  You: I need something fresh and easier on the stomach. Could you please look up some options? I'm finding it hard to think about it.

In this scenario, you are asking your other half to do the practical task of make food *and* you are asking them to take ownership of the mental load of figuring out what. They came up with a solution (pizza) but this does not fit with what you need. You may feel demanding if your partner does not often cook. This dials up the consideration of their discomfort and minimizes your own physical and emotional discomfort in feeling unwell. This is an imbalance, and it is OK to ask more of loved ones when you have less capacity. When you both have reduced capacity, negotiate balance between you – don't default to self-subjugation.

- **Your friends have planned to go to a restaurant that is over-stimulating and makes it difficult to have a conversation, so the evening tends to revolve around alcohol, but you don't want to drink.**
  You [in group chat]: Hey guys, I know you're all keen to go to xxxx but I don't really have a good time there as it is so loud and hard to talk. I really want to properly catch up and hear what's been going on. I'm also not drinking. Can I find some other options?

In this scenario, you are vocalizing the difficulties you have with the chosen venue and highlighting what you want out of the evening, which may well align with what they want too. You are also offering an alternative, so you are not simply saying 'no, pick somewhere else to suit me', making it a fair exchange. Although the rest of the group may have been happy to go to this venue, part of the contract in friendship is about negotiating joint enjoyment and comfort. If they can be comfortable in another venue, while you cannot be comfortable in the chosen one, it makes sense to switch venue. When you are finding alternatives, you will also be considering their comfort.

Dealing with criticism

When you are criticized, your 'emotional' brain regions take over and you can revert to basic fight, flight or freeze instincts that see you being passive, passive-aggressive or aggressive in your response. Responding assertively often isn't intuitive. It is something that you have to practise. Here's how.

1. Write down situations where you feared or experienced criticism. What will people say to you? Why does that worry you? What would the consequences be?
2. Run through one of the situations in your mind, imagining it. It may feel upsetting but it is important so that your body doesn't default to threat mode.
3. When imagining the situation, come up with what you might say to respond to that criticism that feels empowering. Play with wording. Use the guidance from table 13 and the examples just given.
4. Now practise saying it out loud. Repeat this process for the same imagined situation and others if relevant. This helps your body habituate to assertive expression when threatened.

Watch your tone (and body)

Beyond finding the right words, you need to find the right tone. Without practising out loud, it can be hard to get it right in the moment. Keep your tone light, warm and friendly. It helps to try and keep your breathing even, allow yourself pauses and come back to eye contact when you can, rather than looking down, away or past the other person. Although naturally you may find yourself fidgeting, practise trying to be still, shoulders back and head up. Maintain your pitch and volume level.

Practise

Voice out loud the examples in this chapter and experiment with your tone. Pay attention to how your body feels and ground yourself as you go. Repetition helps.

When you are still unheard

You may be reluctant to share feelings or preferences because you're certain that you'll be dismissed or criticized. You may have lots of experience of not being heard or, worse, being punished for sharing your needs. Punishment isn't always overt criticism or harsh words. Sometimes it is a withdrawal of support or affection. The silent treatment, 'ghosting' or pointed changes of the subject, are examples of this. As horrible as this can feel, it doesn't mean your efforts to be assertive are futile. Not when you consider that the alternative is passively allowing the erosion of your right to be heard and to be respected.

When you have expressed yourself clearly and fairly, and others still don't hear you, your story does not end there. Next time this situation or another one like it comes up and you stand by yourself, by practising assertiveness and aiming for equality, you change something. You change something in yourself, and you change something for the person on the other side. Whether or not they explicitly express or act on this change, they have encountered your ability to make a boundary and stand by it. Sometimes it takes multiple rounds of boundary-making being tested, but eventually dynamics shift. In the meantime, you are building courage in yourself, and courage is a powerful force.[*]

---

[*]It is important to consider your capacity. It can take a lot out of you to practise assertiveness, especially where this may be likely to result in

Finding your tribe

One of the biggest protectors against allostatic load and regulators of bodily balance is social support and connection.[61,62,63] Despite the staggering impact on health, the importance of having socially supportive networks is often overlooked at a societal level and, consequently, at an individual level too. Community is garnered through access to free spaces and governmental funding, and requires participation from people who have free time to invest in hobbies and social connection. Unfortunately, this can mean that finding community in modern Western society is not always easy or as happenstance as it used to be.

Some people are lucky enough to be born into families who nail the unconditional love and positive regard. Others stumble into fulfilling friendships. However, for many this is not the case. You acclimatize to the interpersonal culture around you. These cultures may be hostile or insecure, implicitly or explicitly threatening exclusion or rejection. When you acclimatize to these cultures, your brain tends to assume that you are the problem (as explored earlier), rather than the social group you are in. It can feel unsafe to recognize the flaws or failings of your family or friends because the risk is that you'll be left alone.

When my clients and I identify significant social threats that exist in their relationships and social group dynamics, the next course of action is rarely to cut the hostile or insecure attachment loose. Although that may be a decision they come to, it is a big one. Instead, the emphasis is on ensuring that they have sufficient safe relationships and social connection.

This may involve intentionally seeking people and groups that make you feel welcomed as you are, nourish you and align with

---

conflict. Give yourself permission to choose when and who you will practise with – you don't always have to be assertive.

your values. However, research shows that receiving compliments and friendly words of encouragement or affection can feel massively *uncomfortable* if you have never been given a foundation for it feeling safe.[64] If you have not grown up with lots of nourishing social experiences and secure attachment, you have an additional barrier to 'finding your tribe'. You must also train your body to safely receive outward expressions of warmth. I'm not necessarily talking hugs and kisses here. I'm talking about warm words, happy smiles, and explicit sentiments about enjoying seeing you or spending time with you.

Here are some things to consider when setting the intention to have more socially safe experiences and increase social connection:

- **Shared participation and enjoyment**
  Actively engaging in a shared pursuit with others can synchronize neural activity, activating brain reward pathways and stimulating the release of the 'bonding neuropeptide', oxytocin, which reinforces pleasurable sensations and feelings of social connection.[65,66] What shared activities, hobbies or pleasure could you have with your existing network or potentially with others you've yet to meet?

- **Different social support experiences**
  Different people and groups can support different social needs. You may have plenty of people to call for practical support, but not so many for emotional or companionship support. Explore options for different social needs (Figure 26).

- **Patiently cultivate connections**
  If you realize you have had an attrition of close friendships, allow yourself time to explore new avenues for friendship and

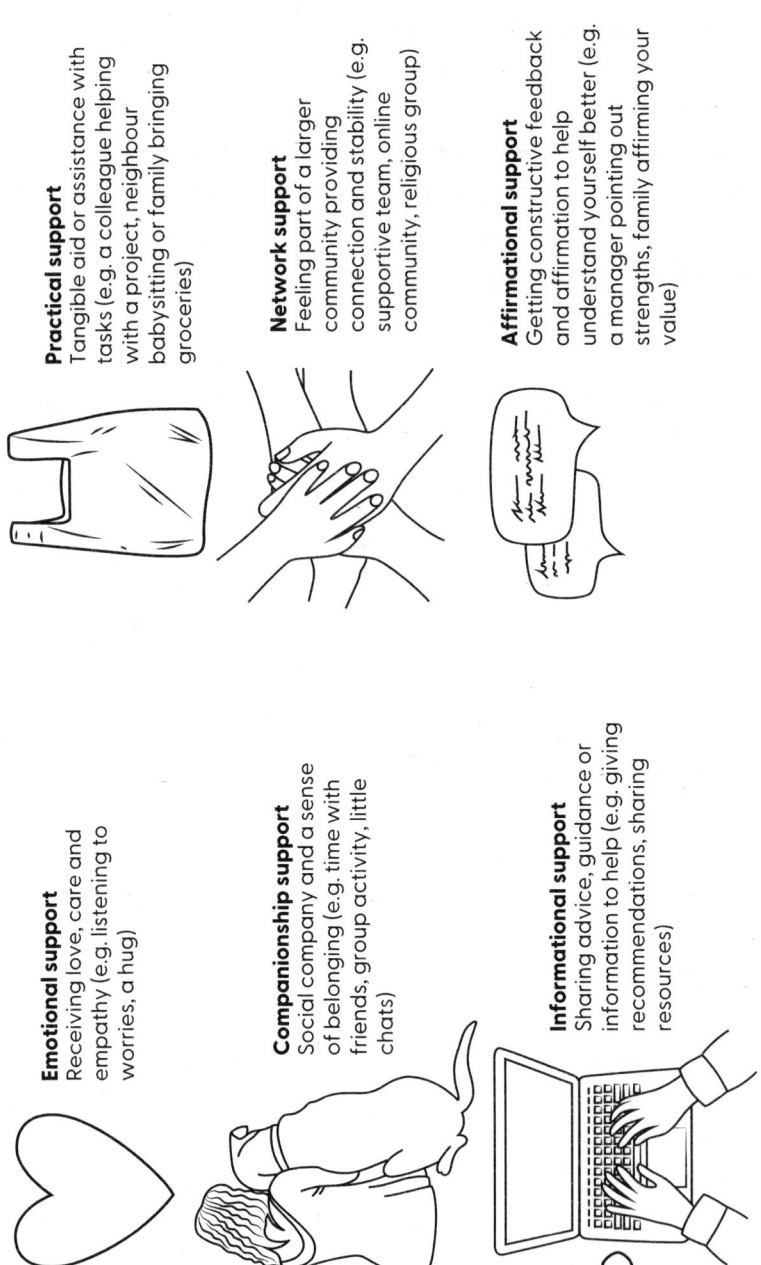

Figure 26: Social support types.

connection. It may feel uncomfortable to begin with, but be explorative, patient and curious.

- **Be intentional.**
  Building new networks requires effort and that requires intention. Map out options for building connection and support using Figure 26. Do your research and then set an intention to make a specific action towards cultivating new connections each week, e.g. joining/attending a new club, suggesting a meet-up, opening a conversation or getting back in touch with an old connection.

Decentring your self

When you are hurting or dealing with lots of stress, your brain sees an increase in activity in areas that are centred around your concept of 'self'. Your brain increases self-focus to protect you. This is not to be confused with selfishness or self-absorption, which are critical phrases your inner-critic may weaponize against you. Increased self-focus amplifies internal threats (thoughts, sensations, emotions), obscuring the external (e.g. the company you are in, what is happening around you). The external is filtered through a lens of self-related threats: Are you being a burden? Have you let them down? This fuels psychobiological loops and disconnection. Clients of mine have been immensely relieved to discover that they can train their brains to do something different. That they can move this attentional spotlight externally when symptomatic and when socially anxious (page 163). This reduces anxiety and makes it easier to sustain conversation, reducing self-consciousness.[67]

Researchers and clinicians alike have observed the healing power of orienting compassionate focus externally towards others, even in the most severe of health challenges. Stephen Porges, creator of polyvagal theory, reflects in his paper, 'A Science of Safety', about how people he observed surviving immense trauma and health issues had an immense sense of connectedness.[68] This shifted them from 'self-focussed survival' to sincere 'actions of compassion, benevolence and generosity'. When I read this paper, I immediately thought of my client Helena. She originally came to me for post-surgery rehabilitation support. She was a delight to work with, lighting up my Mondays with her bright disposition and zany fashion, until one day she shared the news that she had a terminal diagnosis. She asked me if I would continue working with her until the end. From that moment to the very end, our work in therapy was as much about others as it was about helping her to make peace with her fate. I'll never forget the last call we had from her hospice. Zany clothes replaced by hospital gowns and a blanket, her bright disposition remained. She told me, tears of joy in her eyes, how she had managed to mend a long-held conflict with her brother, an act I knew was purely selfless. She did not want him to go on suffering in life while she was at rest in death.

A threatened brain can convince you that you need to focus on defending yourself at the cost of important and healing connection. This is an intuitive sense, but inaccurate.

Compassion practices

You may have heard of the term 'compassion fatigue'. It describes the burnout that can come from extending a lot of care and empathy for others. At some point, you run out of capacity to care so deeply, and this can mean you numb out, feel irritated, withdraw or experience a high degree of overwhelm.

Yet research suggests this shouldn't be called 'compassion' fatigue at all. According to a fascinating study that put a monk in a brain scanner and asked him to practise compassion, it should instead be called 'empathy fatigue'. The monk's name was Matthieu Ricard, a former molecular geneticist who went on to be called 'The Happiest Man in the world' after his participation in another neuroscience study.[69] During that study, he was wired up to 256 sensors which showed that his brain produced gamma waves (associated with consciousness, attention, learning, and memory) at a rate that had never been seen before. There was significant activity in his left PFC, an area linked to positive emotions, suggesting an enhanced capacity for happiness and a diminished tendency toward negativity.

In this subsequent study, the researchers wanted to better understand compassion.[70] However, after a while of Ricard doing his compassion meditation in the brain scanner, they asked him to stop and tell them what precisely he was doing. The activity in his brain did not match the activity in areas of the brain of others when practising compassion. He told them that he was holding others in his mind and sending well wishes and feelings of love towards them. They gave him instructions to instead hold in mind the suffering of others. He complied but this time *he* was eager to stop the meditation. He felt overwhelmed with an urge to escape. Sure enough, the brain activity replicated the patterns of others practising 'compassion'.

This led them to conclude that people mistake empathy for compassion. Empathy is one component of compassion, but not the full picture. Further exploration of brain scan activity helped researchers to clarify the difference between empathy and compassion. Empathy is to experience others' suffering with them, increasing the experience of negative emotions. It also activates areas of the brain that are self-focussed. With empathy there is no differentiation between the self and others' suffering, creating distress, burnout and an inclination to withdraw.

In contrast, compassion is a benevolent sense of warmth and well-wishing, centred around the *motivation* to help not the helplessness arising from limitations in being able to do so. In compassion, social connection, affiliation and unity are elicited and the focus is on the warmth towards others. In follow-up experimentation, researchers found consistent depleting effects of empathy with areas of the brain associated with distress, the self and withdrawal when compared with compassion training, which increased a sense of wellbeing and connection reflected in the brain areas activated.[71]

Replenishing compassion*

You can use the guidance below or the linked audio practice.

Cultivating compassionate feelings

Carve out intentional time to cultivate feelings of warmth towards others. This practice doesn't have to be long, and it doesn't have to involve action. It can be holding a loved one in mind and thinking about their happiness, their successes and their vulnerabilities with affection. As you do, turn towards the experience of warmth and connection you feel for the other/s you are directing your compassion towards.

You may like to start with a pet or child, whose innocence and unconditional love tend to give rise to less complicated feelings that can cloud the practice in other relationships.

Embodying compassionate action

You can embody compassionate action regularly each day no matter your health. List out ways that are accessible to you to foster a sense of compassion regularly in your day-to-day.

Sending a thoughtful text, writing a letter, leaving a voice message, giving someone a compliment, smiling at someone in the street, humanizing those that are often dehumanized (like those begging) by talking to them or simply explaining that you can't give them your charity today. All these little acts are subtle ways of building compassion and a sense of connection.

---

* Download the audio guidance at www.healthpsychologist.co.uk/itsall inyourbody

Transcendence

Compassion and social connection are highly protective experiences. They enhance your sense of interconnection in a world that increasingly feels siloed and individualistic.

In individualistic cultures, pursuits that feed a sense of transcendence are often deprioritized. According to the American Psychological Association (APA), self-transcendence is 'the state in which an individual is able to look beyond himself or herself and adopt a larger perspective that includes concern for others'.[72] Psychologists developed a questionnaire to measure self-transcendence which includes statements like 'my life is meaningful because I live for something greater than myself', 'I focus on discovering the potential meaning in every situation', 'what matters most to me in life is the contribution I make to society'.[73] Inherent in these items is a sense of a greater meaning beyond what is happening to you in any given moment.

When it feels like you are trying to simply survive your day-to-day, pursuits of transcendence can feel like a fanciful privilege reserved for others who have the basics covered. However, research shows that self-transcendence is the biggest protective factor against acting on suicidal thoughts in experiences of extreme crisis.[74] Just how protective self-transcendence can be in adversity was further demonstrated by a study that looked at the impact of the COVID-19 pandemic on mental health. During this time, people were stripped of jobs, roles in their family and social group, and routine, whilst being confronted with death and mortality. Researchers found that those who experienced less negative mental health effects of the pandemic, and adjusted to the difficulties faced, were protected by their capacity for transcendence.

Self-transcendence can be cultivated to hold you in times of difficulty and beyond. Table 14 suggests options to cultivate it.

Benefits of self-transcendence can be obscured by critical

Table 14: Self-transcendent pursuits	
Self-transcendence areas of pursuit	**Description**
Spirituality or religion	Theist religions like Catholicism or Islam can provide self-transcendence. Spirituality can be experienced agnostically or atheistically, by tapping into a sense of something sacred beyond the day-to-day, e.g. an appreciation of nature, creativity, art, philosophy. Star-gazing, forest bathing, attending art exhibitions or music concerts can be self-transcendent experiences.
Awe-seeking	Awe is a self-transcendent emotional response often elicited by a sense of vastness or otherness. Moment-to-moment experiences can arouse this if you attune to them like appreciating a sunset.
Altruistic and prosocial behaviour	Altruism is the desire to increase another's wellbeing. Prosocial behaviour to that effect can follow. Altruism does not have to involve subjugating your own needs. For example, writing a thoughtful card or letter to a friend or family member, or picking up bits of litter in your local park as you walk. Volunteering and altruistic pursuits have cumulative benefits on health.[72]
Collective action	When you feel small or insignificant in your plight, uniting with others who experience the same struggles or are committed to bettering the experience for those like you who are affected, can bring a sense of unity, connection and empowerment, e.g. awareness-raising, fundraising, protesting and group initiatives.

thinking or high expectations. I've had clients who have volunteered, finding catharsis in joining with others to look after vulnerable members of their community, only to start criticizing themselves for not being grateful enough. You can see how your brain itches not only to centre yourself but to tell yourself you are doing something wrong. We'll explore this tendency more in the next chapter.

Principles to extract the benefits of self-transcendence:

- Cultivate the capacity to hold opposing ideas or emotions with creativity and balance, seeking harmony rather than choosing sides. This mindset fosters flexibility, emotional agility, and greater wellbeing. This sees you be able to say, 'They are hugely grateful for the small privilege of a hot meal and I'm struggling to feel grateful for having easy access to hot meals and a house. It feels good to be able to facilitate that feeling in someone else when I cannot easily access it myself.'
- Drop the need for certainty. You don't have to be sure that you've found the 'correct' meaning or you're doing the 'best' thing you could be doing for your common human. It is enough to be intentional.
- Apply savouring (page 190). Lean into the safety, comfort and harmonious feelings that come from engaging in self-transcendent activities.

For your loved ones

I sometimes invite the significant people in my clients' lives into sessions. This may be partners, parents or close friends. The intention is always to enhance connection and collaboration not, as some of my clients have nervously checked with me, to give a telling-off. Loving someone who is suffering is painful and there is no manual in how to best approach it. Having someone external, with a particular framework to explain things, can feel stabilizing for my clients and their loved ones, offering a new way to approach old ruts or contentions.

I created the next section to be handed to the people of significance in your life, so that they may feel better supported to support you, and aided to look after themselves. It might be something you read together, or something you read and take ideas from to discuss. Whatever you decide, it is important to know that it is not all on your shoulders.

You've been passed this page by a person who trusts you with it. The fact that it feels safe enough to pass you this page, means that you are already a hugely restorative force in their life. You've been passed this page because someone you care for deeply is dealing with something complicated and that means that you are too.

When you are supporting someone to heal or to manage something not easily healable or unhealable, it can be incredibly difficult for you both. The person you are supporting has read the rest of this book to this point, so they are equipped with knowledge and insight that may make that a bit easier. Now it's time to give you some guidance so that you may be united in your efforts together. The intention is for you both to feel empowered as a team.

Your cup

Don't pour from an empty cup. Caring for someone dealing with adversity in whatever capacity you are caring for them, will deplete you if you don't attend to your own mental and physical health. Prioritize that, it's important.

Your shared cup

Looking after your mental and physical health isn't automatically at odds with supporting your loved one. Organizing times to connect, explore, enjoy and reflect can simultaneously fill your cups. These don't have to be big things; picking a film you both enjoy, cooking together, getting outside in beautiful scenery. These moments are truly restorative psychologically and physiologically.

Same page

One of the biggest causes of relational tension and stress in chronic illness is having different understandings of what is happening, why it is happening and what needs to happen. In illness, the human brain likes to simplify and point to as few causes and solutions as possible. For example, 'your symptoms are worse when you're anxious, so your anxiety is causing your symptoms', or 'your mood is lower when you go to work, so you should find a new job'. Although not necessarily incorrect, the simplicity can overlook important complexity that leaves the person having the experience feeling misunderstood. You don't have to agree on everything but having a shared understanding of their experience is important. This is an invitation for you to explore with your loved one whether you have a shared understanding of what contributed to the difficulties they are facing, what keeps them going and what will help. If you are up for it, set a time to initiate this conversation. Chapter 1 can help.

Hearing before fixing

Because it is so hard to see someone you care for suffer, your brain tries to find fixes. This is important and, in many ways, helpful, but finding a fix is not always the solution. Instead, making someone feel heard has the power to soothe distress and even physiological dysregulation.[75,76,77]

When you are inclined to make suggestions of what might help, be sure to pause first. Instead of looking for or suggesting a fix, focus on making them feel heard by acknowledging and asking questions, such as, 'You're going through so much. Is there anything I can do to help?' Or, 'I can see you're overwhelmed. Would you like me to make some suggestions?' Work on recognizing and accepting when your loved one doesn't have the capacity to work on solutions right away.

Trigger traps

People experience lots of social stigma when impacted by illness and/or mood difficulties. This comes in the form of being disbelieved, discredited, perceived as weak or failing and being excluded or rejected. Not all these experiences are super obvious to the outside world but they are incredibly painful if you are the one experiencing them. This means your brain becomes physically primed to expect these social threats and easily triggered to respond emotionally when detected. You may have found yourself on the receiving end of emotional outbursts. This is hard for you and for your loved one. Try and navigate these moments with respect (for yourself and your loved one) and compassion. You don't have to 'take it', but equally don't amplify the emotional heat by engaging strong defences or attacking back. When you both can, explore options for navigating communication in areas that most commonly lead to difficult interactions. It is a joint effort for you both to feel safe with each other.

Common trigger points in communication involve sentiments that can be construed to mean your loved one is:

- Not trying hard enough to improve things
- Over-exaggerating or making things up
- Going to be left on their own or excluded.

You may find trigger situations are diffused by expressly communicating the opposite, such as, 'I know how hard you are trying' or 'I can see how much you're hurting' or 'I'm here for you'.

You were passed these pages, to help your loved one recognize that their healing is not all on them and to reduce their internal pressure. Equally their healing is not all on you. You and your loved one might find it useful to use Figure 27 to explore how you may collectively look after each other.

In this chapter you've learnt:

- The biology of your inbuilt social barometer and how it detects for social threats and cues of safety
- The automatic evolutionarily ingrained biological responses to social threats

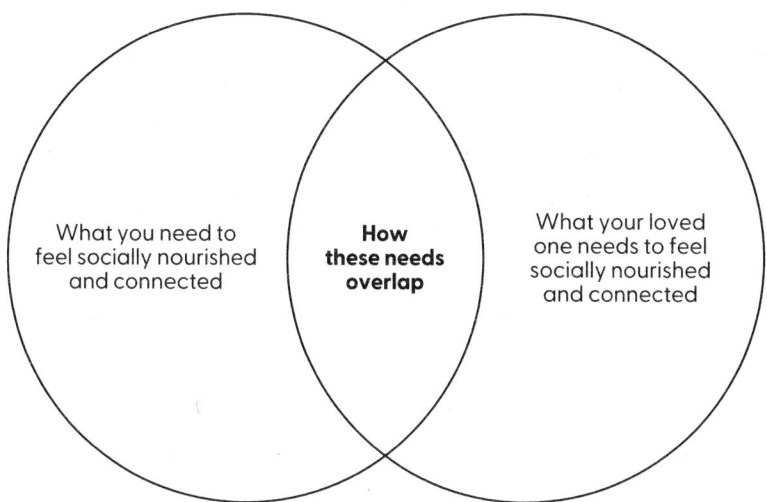

Figure 27: A template for you and your loved one(s) to explore social nourishment and connection needs.

- How various societal injuries can impact your health, including gender discrimination, racism, ageism and ableism
- Steps for increasing social safety including self-advocacy and assertiveness, building social connection, self-transcendence and compassion.

Throughout this book I've described experiences of feeling totally misunderstood and unheard by those closest to me and experiences of feeling utterly seen and supported.

These experiences have had profound impacts on me in their own ways. I'll never forget the pain of being misunderstood and mistreated when I was at my most vulnerable (in many experiences I haven't included in this book). And the pain of owning that pain, as though it was my fault or because of an internal deficit that would render me perpetually powerless. I hope this chapter helped you to better recognize that responsibility for your vulnerability or depletion is not yours to own.

Self-growth and healing are topics that are rarely considered in the context of social connection and the world around you.

Narratives instead focus on solo defeats of adversity. We seldom hear stories glorifying the power of connection and the healing that can be unlocked by its prioritization. And yet, in groups that I've run and in the online community I host, the transformative essence of social connection is clear. Many of the members of my online community have experienced the social threats we have considered in this chapter, often very severely and repeatedly. And yet, with a curious, open spirit and a little hope, they have chosen to open Zoom to meet with a bunch of strangers towards a common goal of befriending their bodies. In so doing, they have cultivated a strong, safe and beautiful community ready to listen and to work together.

In finishing the writing of this chapter, I had to cancel one of the evening workshops last-minute. A long day, after a series of long days, sat in a beanbag while writing on a laptop, had resulted in migraine. As I messaged the group to apologize for any disappointment, two wonderful things happened. The first: I was greeted with an abundance of messages of good will and encouragement, saying, 'Don't be sorry, you are practising what you preach', and 'Look after yourself, Dr Sula.' I felt the warmth in my chest as the sentiments radiated from the phone. The second: one of the group members opened the suggestion of meeting anyway, to collectively explore what they had been working on. More messages flooded in enthusiastically coordinating how to do this. Unable to look at my phone any longer, the migraine kicking up, another feeling welled up and brought tears to my eyes. There isn't a word for this feeling. But it was wholesome, warming and utterly reassuring. It was the beauty of knowing that these people were looking out for each other. That at the moment I was resting my head on my pillow, they were sharing their thoughts and feelings safely with each other towards the common aim of healing.

Rest assured, if you have not found your safe community yet, it is out there. Use this chapter to create some stepping-stone goals (page 25) to help you cultivate more social safety. It truly matters, as do you.

SECTION THREE

Sustaining change and becoming who you are

'I wouldn't choose to have this, but I'm grateful for how it has changed me'
– CLIENT REFLECTING ON CHRONIC ILLNESS JOURNEY

How are you feeling now? Have you been trying things out or are you mulling things over, deciding what to prioritize? My work with clients incorporates the information and practices in the last two sections. When clients feel shifts in their mind–body relationship, it can be a case of simply repeating and varying practices. However, for many others I work with, this is just the starting point.

Years of just coping, being on guard against your own biology and withstanding societal hardships, can permeate on a deeper level. A deeper level that affects how you see yourself. If you are to sustain the changes from previous chapters, you need to claim compassionate ownership of yourself, recognizing what you value about yourself and what you want to value.

This is precisely what we will explore in the coming chapters. All the reading (and work) you have done to this point will allow you to more easily recognize and engage with the concepts and practices in these chapters. In turn this will support you to sustain the changes you have been making so far (even if just conceptual at this point). This is not easy work, but it is important. Give yourself grace to explore with a light touch and curiosity and see what comes of it.

In the final section we're going to cover:

- What beliefs are, how they are programmed and how they affect your health
- Why and how to change your beliefs for the good of your health
- How to reclaim your sense of self and build confidence in your own worth
- How to define and live by your values so that they can sustain you in sickness and in health.

CHAPTER 8

Updating your beliefs

You've had a window into moments of my illness, from the time I careered out of the house in utter overwhelm to the dismay of my dad, to the times I spent meditating beside him. These were belief-forming, crystallizing moments. When I first became unwell, many of my experiences suggested that I would not recover or ever feel better. The rapid development of this belief created a lot of despair that fed many symptom spirals, fuelling more fearful thoughts, overwhelming emotions and heightened physical symptoms.

The idea of 'I will never feel better' seemed less of a belief and more of a knowledge when I was tethered to the toilet at my dad's little cottage. Less than a year later, I'd be interviewing for the health psychology master's at King's College London, full of hope and barely symptomatic. You may think that what updated the belief from 'I'll never feel better' to 'things can be OK' was symptoms receding. The thing is, my beliefs started to shift before my symptoms reduced. You may recall two of these belief-shifting moments in this book: one, where my dad's partner, a clinical psychologist, helped me better understand how my body was working (page 108); the other, when I practised mindfulness with my dad and experienced a different way of being with my mind and body (page 193). Although not solid proof that things would work out, they offered choices and hope. Enough for me to start interrupting symptom spirals and feel just a little different. Enough to ease my body closer to balance so that it could start healing.

This is the thing about beliefs. They have an incredible amount of power in determining our experience of a moment and the potential of future moments. Psychosocially constructed and biologically encoded, beliefs can impact your health directly psychobiologically and indirectly through your behaviours. Throughout life you will accumulate many beliefs, some standing firm and enduring, others more flexible, acquiescent to change. Some of these beliefs will more directly determine your health and these are the beliefs that require examination and (potentially) updating to aid your healing goals.

In this chapter, you will become acquainted with your own belief systems and how they may help or hinder your healing journey. Your belief systems are a reflection of the cultures you have been exposed to, the family environment you grew up in and the experiences you have had. All these things shape you, but they don't *determine* you. On this task, we're going to look at the scope for updating long-held beliefs that keep you stuck, scared or resigned, using neuroscience and trauma therapy principles to work with, not against, your brain.

Health-altering beliefs

In Chapter 6, you were introduced to beliefs as deeply ingrained ideas shaped by repetitive experiences and thoughts. If thoughts arise from electrical and chemical signalling between neurons, then beliefs are the result of synaptic connections being reinforced over time, forming ready-made neural networks that help you navigate the world. The phrase 'neurons that fire together, wire together' reflects how repeated activation of certain neural pathways strengthens their connections. The more frequently your experiences activate specific neurons, the stronger and more efficient their connections become. Over time, these reinforced pathways coalesce into stable neural networks, shaping and embedding beliefs.

Beliefs can be formed in all shapes and sizes, from simple to more complex. They are often experienced as knowledge, although they are not necessarily true. Have you had moments where you've been corrected about something you could have sworn was fact? This could be matters of trivia you assumed you knew or personal recollections (e.g. how events unfolded). When (if) you realize you were incorrect, this is a moment of a belief masquerading as knowledge. That sense of knowledge or truth is important. It relates to the experience explored in Chapter 5, of being caught between 'head' and 'heart'. Long-held beliefs can make you feel one way, when information you are receiving or an experience you are having tells you something else. For example, a doctor may tell you a procedure will be safe and has the statistics to back it up. However, an underlying belief of 'you can't trust doctors', informed by many prior highly distressing experiences, will make it hard for you to believe the statistics. Your underlying belief feels truer and so you will use it to guide your actions.

Beliefs with the biggest effect on your health are 'health beliefs' and 'core beliefs'. Health beliefs are beliefs specifically related to your health and health behaviours. Core beliefs are a concept from cognitive psychotherapy. According to this model of therapy and supported by neurodevelopmental disciplines, you have core beliefs about yourself (e.g. I am a good person/I am a bad person), others (e.g. people are kind/people can't be trusted) and the world (e.g. the world is safe/the world is hostile). Core beliefs are the building blocks you start with to understand yourself and your place in the world. Generally, people develop an array of core beliefs – positive, negative and neutral. Although it follows that negative experiences can create negative core beliefs and positive experiences can create positive core beliefs, often there is more nuance. We'll explore the development of these beliefs in a moment.

Health beliefs

Two widely researched health psychology models explain just how much of an impact health beliefs have on your health experiences.[1,2] Figure 28 combines insights from these models. It illustrates how early life experiences form broad beliefs about health, thereby influencing the development of specific illness beliefs when you become

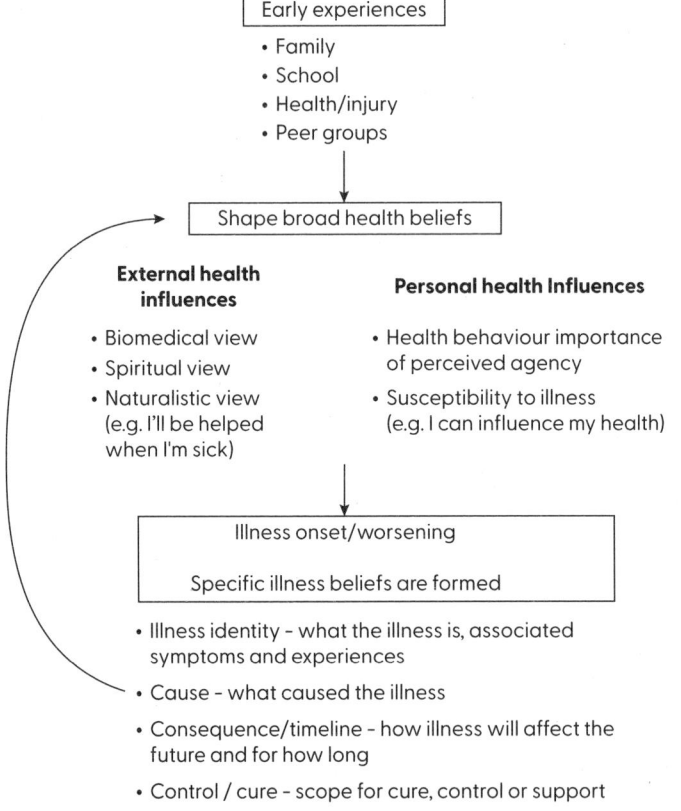

Figure 28: Broad beliefs about health impact the formation of specific perceptions of illness. This illustration combines concepts from the health belief model and the illness representation model.

ill or when your health declines. Broad beliefs about the external influences of health are culturally informed, such as whether you believe illness is caused by pathogens, a God, or naturalistic forces.[3] I've had clients who believe their ailments are due to karma or a curse, which had a huge impact on how we approached generating a sense of personal agency.

Broad beliefs about personal influence over health will be heavily informed by your past experiences. As we've explored, a diminished sense of personal control is psychobiologically threatening, as is an over-inflated sense of responsibility.

Simply put, unconsciously held beliefs about health will have a very significant impact when you become ill, potentially breeding a lot of self-stigma, blame or sense of powerlessness. People who sense that illness is a karmic punishment may feel confused and guilty when they get ill, worrying they did something to deserve it. Those who believe Western medicine is toxic will feel fearful when their condition deteriorates, believing treatment options are damaging and therefore not an option. As well as influencing what you do (your health behaviours) and how you feel, health beliefs and specific illness perceptions can alter your physiological bodily processes, as we considered earlier in relation to the placebo/nocebo effect (page 217).[4]

At the beginning of this book, I invited you to engage with an approach to health that is broader than the traditional biomedical view: a biopsychosocial view. In doing so, I was inviting you to consciously shape your own broad health beliefs, with the potential to adjust negative core beliefs. The societal message 'it's all in your head' infers that it's your responsibility to heal, you're on your own to heal and you can't trust yourself or your body. These sentiments can influence core beliefs of being weak, defective, insignificant and more. We'll explore core beliefs further in a moment.

I've gradually introduced you to more data, research and anecdote to help shift away from beliefs like these and explore the basis for alternative safer beliefs and how they might work in practice.

Now I'm going to make the invitation even more explicit, by presenting you with the impact of adopting biopsychosocial health beliefs versus viewing health as purely biomedical. A purely biomedical view of health sees you as an organism with complex biology that can go awry. When it does, it requires biomedical intervention, of which you are a passive recipient. Often, an overly restrictive and inflexible biomedical approach overlooks the interconnectivity of the body (e.g. how brain processing can impact your heart or gut) and if it does acknowledge the interconnectivity, with a view to offset the side effects of treatments, its significance can be downplayed, which can feel disconcerting. Inherent to this approach is a power dynamic between patient and practitioner. The patient's experiences of health are viewed as less important than the 'objective' metrics of the average success of procedures.[5] This is why patients can be turned away for further treatment or investigation, even though they still have severely intrusive symptoms.

In contrast, a biopsychosocial view of health sees biomedical intervention as a potentially fundamental part of recovery (or health maintenance) alongside non-medical support and personal agency. Biopsychosocial approaches to health emphasize the importance of collaboration in healthcare consultations, with informed choice and empathetic communication. Your support networks are viewed as powerful in their propensity to aid your recovery practically and emotionally. This approach gives you agency, flexibility and recognizes your humanity.

I invite you to adopt a biopsychosocial view of health, recognizing that it has the potential to alter multiple downstream illness perceptions (Figure 28), and ultimately your health. In learning just how much your psychological and social experiences impact health, although you may have always suspected it, you are now armed with specific ways to enact that influence. Experimenting with that influence creates empowering experiences, leading to improvements in your health. Previous chapters have demonstrated how brain activity can physically change processes in your body with a direct impact on health and bodily balance. There is much research demonstrating how significantly perceptions of illness impact illness trajectories, such as determining things like hospital readmission, returning to work after illness, degree of disability, pain and fatigue.[6,7] If, having read to this point, you feel pretty convinced that there are psychosocial avenues that can positively influence your health, chances are that your brain and body are already running processes in the background to help you engage with those influences. That's powerful!

Core beliefs

Core beliefs also have huge significance for your biological bodily processes and overall health. They determine a lot of what you think, feel, and do, as well as your physiology. They can be considered the iceberg underpinning much of your present-moment experiences, and therefore also fuelling symptom spirals. A neutral core belief of 'I'm athletic' will likely drive motivation and engagement with exercise, influencing your physical fitness, weight, cardiovascular health, and so on. This belief may also have negative consequences if it leads to complacency, meaning that you don't challenge yourself physically and your health suffers; or if your athleticism is compromised and then you feel that this element of who you are is lost. The reality is that many positive, negative or neutral core beliefs can exert multiple effects on a continuum from beneficial to unhelpful. To fully consider the impact of core beliefs and, importantly, how you can update them for your mental and physical wellbeing, you need to understand how they are formed.

Why do you believe that?

The last chapter described different ways that your social world can shape you. Your brain constantly sifts through sensory information to understand yourself, others and the world around you as it has evolved to do for survival. We've explored how, according to polyvagal theory and compassion-focussed therapy, your physiology is designed to help determine social as well as physical safety.[8,9] You have seen throughout these chapters how your body has ways to determine this from the 'bottom up' (i.e. the body sending messages to the brain) and from the 'top down' (i.e. cognitive processes in the brain to the body). Both pathways work together to combine data during multisensory integration (Chapter 3).

In your early years, much of your sense of safety is determined by how safe you feel emotionally and physiologically, because much of your brain has yet to fully form, with a vast number of synaptic connections pending. As you start to form more sophisticated cognitive processing, beliefs in development are hugely informed by how safe you have felt preverbally as a young infant.[10]

This does not mean that your baby-to-toddlerhood years are always the *primary* influencers of how you come to later think about things, but they do create your foundational template for later thought development, both in terms of what you come to think and how you are *able* to think.

In your development, you have 'critical periods' where your brain is particularly malleable to input from your surroundings, which will shape future brain processing. There are critical periods throughout your early development for forming secure attachments with others, learning social behaviours, developing your identity and higher cognitive functions like reasoning and planning. Middle childhood to adolescence (from 6 years old to 18 years old) is a critical period for social development and higher cognitive functions. Your brain and bodily biology is spongelike, ready to absorb and hold your experiences. How you are talked to, treated, your physical experiences, what you witness, will all have a big impact on how you form your own beliefs about yourself, others and the world.

Research shows that your inner voice (the dialogue you

experience in your head) is heavily shaped by the words, tone and style of primary caregivers in your early life.[11] If you were often corrected, told you were being silly, told 'it's not possible', you are much more likely to have an inner voice that reflects this. Similarly, in later childhood and adolescence, witnessing how your parents, grandparents and siblings figure things out and deal with problems, informs how you approach problem-solving. In my work with clients, there is a high tendency for rumination and worry. Often when exploring with clients, we will note that Mum and/or Dad tended to worry out loud, to try and establish fixes and to create contingency plans. This heavily reflects what is often going on in the heads of my clients when faced with problems that aren't easily solvable, getting them stuck in cycles of worry and rumination.

Your cognitive capacity expands, becoming more sophisticated as you grow. You start off processing experiences categorically: good versus bad, happy versus sad, safe versus scary. You can see this in children's books and learning material using categories, like colours and farmyard animals. Nuance and lateral thinking start to expand as categories are merged (e.g. farmyard animals of a particular colour), and then continuums are introduced, from number scales through to colour spectrums. You develop the ability to broaden templates for understanding the world around you and indeed yourself.

Using categories to help process information can be a very efficient way for your brain to make sense of things. How many times have you heard a phrase like 'he's the kind of person who . . .' Depending on what's at the end of this sentence (e.g. 'who votes for Trump' or 'who protests for animal rights'), your brain has a ready-made conceptualization for that person based on the category they've been placed in. Likely you may also have an inference of whether you would get on with them or not. However, too much reliance on a binary way of cognitive processing can be problematic. Labels have power. They can obscure nuance that is important for agency and change. This is illustrated in studies showing that people who receive a label of depression when experiencing milder symptoms of depression, feel less agency over improving their mood.[12] Labels can be limiting in how they affect your perception and emotional state, both of which can maintain symptom spirals, thereby potentially worsening outcomes (page 108 – Chapter 3).

If you're raised in cultures or systems that perpetuate categorical (all-or-nothing) thinking, this is likely to influence the development of rigid beliefs about yourself, the world and others. Let's take schools with a strong emphasis on high performance: although there are grading scales from A* through to F, the way you are treated, what feedback you get, what 'set' you are put in, can make the brain reduce this grading system into 'smart', 'average' and 'stupid'. Many clients of mine have told me how, when getting 95% on a test, the reaction of the school and/or parents would be to enquire about the 5% not done correctly. The implication clearly being that getting less than 100% was not good enough. Explicit messages about worth and acceptability can come in the form of judgements about you *and* witnessing judgements of others. Hearing your mum call the woman down the road a 'hussy' can inform your sense of what a hussy is, what it would mean to be one and how you can avoid that condemnation yourself.

On a neuroscience and biochemical level, beliefs can be reinforced through dopaminergic reward pathways so that thinking a certain way (and acting congruently) produces positive feelings, which subsequently reinforce the belief. You may get a sense of satisfaction for working hard, which reinforces the idea that working really hard is a good thing. Oxytocin, the hormone involved in bonding and social connection, can also increase the likelihood of forming beliefs that align with those you trust and feel a sense of belonging with.[13] When you share experiences with people who have similar symptoms, concerns, and motivations, you may be more inclined to adopt their opinions and judgements about a particular treatment, approach or lifestyle. This implicit trust, fostered by shared experiences, enhances your brain's readiness to form and reinforce neural networks, solidifying these beliefs over time.[14]

Beliefs are biopsychosocially developed and maintained with biopsychosocial repercussions. We will look at how we can use principles from neuroscience and neurobiology to update beliefs that will protect, even enhance, your health and sense of self-worth. First, you need to be able to recognize what you are working with and where updates may be necessary.

Threatening beliefs

Adversity, illness and trauma make the development of 'threatening' beliefs more likely. Threatening beliefs are core and/or health beliefs that make you feel unsafe or vulnerable as you are. They may be related to physical safety (e.g. 'I am vulnerable', 'I have no control') or sense of worth (e.g. 'I'm failing', 'I'm wrong'). Your brain is quick to develop beliefs about things that are of central importance to your survival and safety.

In previous chapters, we considered the experiences you may have when you become ill or suffer adversity: you can't trust yourself, you're on your own, the pressure to get better is all on you. These can become beliefs you internalize because underlying each sentiment are threats to your core safety needs as identified in the power threat meaning framework. Table 15 describes each of these core safety needs, with examples of how threat to these needs may result in the development of threatening beliefs about yourself, others or the world.

The development of threatening beliefs can be considered your brain's way of internalizing external threats so that you can be ready to (theoretically) protect yourself. However, internalized threatening beliefs can keep your body in threat mode. Threat mode sees areas of the brain dedicated to processing threat (amygdala, hippocampus and hypothalamus) activated, which means your attention is attuned to threats, reducing your sense of safety

Table 15: Examples of the development of negative threat beliefs in relation to core safety needs according to the power threat meaning framework

Core need	Threatening experiences example	Example belief formed
Attachment	Parents scold or ignore you when highly distressed	**Self:** I am a burden (when I am upset) **Others:** People will reject me (if I am honest with how I feel) **World:** Vulnerability is bad
Control	School system won't let you go to the toilet when you need to go	**Self:** My body is wrong **Others:** People won't understand **World:** My needs won't be accommodated when I have symptoms
Basic physical and material needs not being met	Having ongoing sickness and not getting answers from doctors	**Self:** I am powerless **Others:** People won't help **World:** The world is uncaring
Sense of fairness and justice	Seeing your sibling cooed over when ill, whilst you are told you are moaning	**Self:** I'm insignificant **Others:** People are more important than me **World:** The world favours the fortunate
Being valued	Being picked last for team activities	**Self:** I am not good enough **Others:** People will not appreciate me **World:** To succeed you must show value
Meaning	Being pushed towards academic work when you have a talent for art and creativity	**Self:** I'm worthless **Others:** People respect intelligence **World:** Art and creativity is an indulgence not an important contribution to society

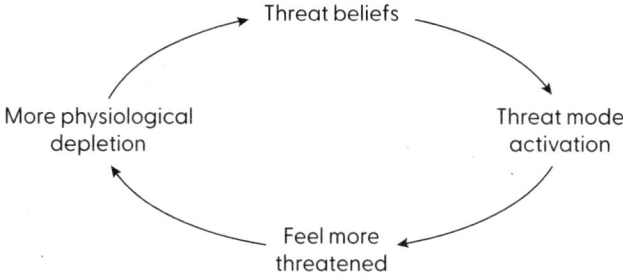

Figure 29: How threat beliefs are maintained and create cycles of bodily depletion contributing to allostatic load.

and ease. It also makes your body more reactive. The more reactive your body is to potential threats, the more demand on your regulatory systems and potentially the more physical (and emotional) discomfort you have. Therefore, paradoxically, threatening beliefs deplete your body and can contribute to allostatic load, making you more vulnerable, which then reinforces existing threat beliefs and potentially creates new ones (Figure 29).

Past trauma and adversity create threatening beliefs that can keep affecting things in the present, as the body (and mind) remains primed to threat. I see a lot of clients who have grown up in comparatively safe environments with secure attachments, but who find it impossible to access that sense of safety once they have started dealing with symptoms of ill-health (mental or physical). Aside from the role of self-criticism (discussed in Chapter 6), one of the reasons for this is the trauma of their reality changing. It is itself devastatingly threatening, to go from believing 'I can be helped when I need it' to 'no one will help me'. Or 'I am safe' to 'I am vulnerable'. I call this 'belief flipping'. When beliefs flip from safe to threat, your brain can question many other assumptions it has had about safety, which can be incredibly destabilizing and lead to ongoing cycles, as depicted in Figure 29.

Developing beliefs for empowerment & safety

In order to stop your body from staying stuck in threat mode and reactive, you have to update your beliefs. The intention in updating beliefs is not to rewrite reality or create your own delusions. People I work with face very real, very difficult problems with accessing treatment they desperately need in the healthcare system. It stands to reason that they have beliefs like 'I cannot be helped' or 'I am powerless'. I am not encouraging them to convince themselves of alternative beliefs like 'I can get help whenever I need it'. That's not going to be convincing and, if it was, it certainly would not be helpful in a context where this will be contradicted quickly. Belief updates should be a more realistic and less threatening alternative that holds space for the grey areas. For example, 'I cannot be helped' may move to something like 'I can find choices'.

Updating beliefs in this way recalibrates your brain from a default position of threat and despair to a more open and safe position. The safer the headspace, the more able the body is to come back to balance and restore (homeostasis). To change your beliefs is to change your neural pathways. You are shifting from one (or many) default pathway to another. The problem is the 'other' new pathway may not exist yet so you have to create it. This task is as exciting as it is perhaps unknowable. Exactly how that process unfolds will be different for everyone, but over the next pages we'll look at how you can help your brain to do just that, even when you are still experiencing symptoms.

Your brain clings to old beliefs

Before you embark on the journey of updating beliefs, it's important you know the strong defences your brain possesses to keep old beliefs in place. You need to know this because when you come up against these defences, they can feel pretty convincing and cause you to conclude that the old threatening beliefs were right all along. You might abandon your efforts, old beliefs intact, keeping body in threat mode and depleted. We don't want this! Here's what you need to know.

Conflicting beliefs are tidied away swiftly

When you become aware that beliefs you have held for a long time may no longer serve you or may be inaccurate, this can create cognitive dissonance. Cognitive dissonance is the discomfort that arises from an internal conflict between your beliefs (and/or behaviours), motivating your brain to reduce the inconsistency. For example, you recognize that avoiding plans makes you feel physically and emotionally worse, but you have an old belief that fears plans (e.g. you'll let people down if you cancel). Your brain's choices are to change your belief (e.g. making plans is beneficial) or to reject or rationalize the contradicting evidence. Your brain is so keen to get rid of the discomfort of conflicting beliefs, it prioritizes speed over precision. Rationalizing or rejecting disconfirming evidence is less metabolically demanding than changing your beliefs. Your brain has a tool to swiftly tidy away belief conflicts.

The brain's tool of choice: cognitive immunization

Cognitive immunization strategies are psychological mechanisms that allow your brain to reject or resist information that contradicts your existing beliefs. Cognitive immunization may involve:

- **Rationalizing away the evidence:** 'The plans made me feel good because I know I had an out'
- **Cherry-picking information:** 'Jerry was angry I cancelled' [ignoring the five friends who were understanding]
- **Reframing the information:** 'I get more anxious when I have plans'

- **Emotional reasoning:** You may remember this from previous chapters – 'I feel safer not making plans'

Nareena's story

These strategies happen quick as a flash and are very convincing, serving to keep old beliefs in place and inhibiting change. I worked with a client, Nareena, who was 40 years old and had held the belief her whole life that it was not OK to feel difficult emotions. In her childhood, she had been told off for crying and appraised as 'difficult' when she felt something intensely. Experiencing emotions intensely felt wrong and, as she often told me in session, 'pointless'. After doing some work together, she knew that this belief was making it harder for her to regulate her emotions and had a role in her recurrent bladder pain flare-ups. No matter how clear she was with me that her goal was to accept her difficult emotions and be able to feel them without pushing them away, there were many sessions where the same sentiments and blocks would come up: 'perhaps it *is* bad to feel these emotions because I feel terrible' or 'it just isn't productive to feel sad'. I have to say, these cognitive immunization expressions were so convincing that I had to keep checking with my supervisor – 'Are we doing the right thing?' – and reflected with Nareena often about whether she still wanted to befriend her emotions and how this related to her therapy goals. When trying to work with changing long-held beliefs, these cognitive defences can be strong and persuasive. They were developed with good reason and have probably *protected* you in lots of ways, even where they have also hurt you. It can be a tough job to convince the brain that it's safe to change them.

One of the most common cognitive immunization examples I hear from clients is this: 'I'm back to square one'. This is a form of cherry-picking and emotional reasoning. I usually hear this after months of my clients implementing things from therapy having resulted in progress towards their stepping-stone goals. A flare-up or knock-back can cause the brain to shout 'you're back to square one' because changing beliefs is so uncomfortable. For a long time, clients may have believed 'there's nothing I can do'. When they start to try out 'I have choices' it feels precarious. At the first sign of doubt, the brain likes to rebound back to the 'safety' of familiar beliefs. That is why when making changes to ingrained beliefs you need to build your tolerance for that discomfort.

Tolerating uncertainty

Not knowing what will happen or whether what you are doing will work can be excruciating. You only have so much capacity to tolerate uncertainty. Some people are more sensitive to uncertainty, which can cause a lot of anxiety and safety behaviours (page 117). You can increase your tolerance of uncertainty to the point that uncertainty can even feel comfortable. The more tolerant to uncertainty, the less distress cognitive dissonance causes and the easier it is to adjust and reinforce new beliefs. You have already been building the skill of tolerating uncertainty through the practice exercises in this book. The ones in Chapters 5 and 6 are particularly relevant. Continue practising to help update your beliefs.

Spotting beliefs to be updated

To update beliefs, you need to first make the unconscious conscious by building metacognitive awareness. We're going to use a similar process to thought-logging (page 204) to help you identify themes of thoughts and behaviours, to trace back to the underlying belief/s.

There are some beliefs that you wear on your sleeve, so to speak, but there are many others that you may have a hard time identifying or even believing you believe them. Lots of my clients are high-earning over-achievers with great accolades. They can acknowledge their strengths and what they have accomplished.

However, they are wracked with anxiety or a sense that it will all go away if they stop working hard. When I pose a question about whether they feel they aren't capable or aren't safe or secure, they may initially dismiss it. 'I *know* I *am capable*. I couldn't have gotten this far if I wasn't!'

This is where I may recap with my clients on the developmental formation of beliefs (page 280). I also often use a conceptualization from internal family systems: you are a complex, multidimensional person. You don't have one way of thinking about yourself. You have different self-concepts and, with that, different modi operandi. There is a part of you that is fiercely capable and has trust in this – perhaps puts too much pressure on you to be capable ('managerial part', page 183). However, there may be a more vulnerable part of you that fears that you aren't inherently capable. This part may fear that you are *just managing* to keep things afloat by using precarious strategies like chronic busyness, tightly controlled schedules or health regimes. If that all goes, the fear may be that you'll be exposed for how incapable you '*actually* are'.

It doesn't always come down to capability. As shown in Table 16, you can have a vast array of beliefs about yourself with various threat considerations. So, how do you spot them if your core beliefs aren't obvious to you? Here are some options.

> **In previous chapters, you were invited to log thoughts as part of symptom spirals (Chapter 3) and building metacognitive awareness (Chapter 6). If you did this, you may like to get your notes out for reference.**
>
> Do you notice any patterns or themes coming up? Beneath these thoughts, your deeper threatening beliefs may be coming to the surface.
>
> It can be easier to recognize the beliefs once you hear them or see them, rather than to try and construct what they are by reading back your thoughts. I created Table 16 to help. You have the choice to identify thoughts you resonate with from the column of examples

> and use the subsequent columns to help you specify potential underlying belief(s). Alternatively, you may consider the threat themes, which are clustered around core safety need threats (page 284) to see which feel most personally relevant. From there you can consider whether any of the related core beliefs – or variations of them – resonate.
>
> At this stage, you're exploring what beliefs may be making your brain and body feel threatened. Before updating the beliefs, it is helpful to reflect on how these beliefs have been feeding a sense of threat in your mind and body. Revisit Chapter 3 to trace out how your beliefs have been influencing your symptom spirals.

When using Table 16, give yourself licence to play around with the phrasing so that it is more tailored to you and your experience. Please note, this table is not exhaustive and is not a precise formula, but more of a guideline. There are many different rules you can develop for one core belief, rather than there being one rule per core belief. You may have multiple rules and core beliefs, and some of them quite likely contradict each other. For example, a rule about always being agreeable, may conflict with a rule about never putting yourself in situations where you feel vulnerable. If someone asks you to a party they are hosting, but you don't know anyone, you may feel torn. It feels like you would be doing something wrong by turning down the invitation, but going feels hugely exposing and scary. When two rules work against each other, it can be a confusing experience that can activate stress processes and threat mode causing you to worry excessively and/or ruminate.

Behaviours betray beliefs

You can also explore whether what you are doing (your behaviours) are giving any clues to what underlying threatening beliefs

Table 16: Commonly experienced thoughts and expectations and related underlying core beliefs

Thought examples	Related rules	Threat themes	Possible core beliefs
Symptoms will get worse The worst thing to happen might happen It won't be OK if things don't go to plan	Always prepare for the worst Don't leave anything to chance Always reduce the risk of things going wrong	Safety	I cannot trust my body I cannot protect myself I'm in danger
People don't care I will be rejected I am behind everyone	Never rely on others Always try your hardest Always be likeable	Self-worth	I am insignificant I am incapable I am worthless I am shameful
I shouldn't have done . . . I should have I might burden them if I . . .	Always prepare for the worst Always be aware of others' feelings and take them into consideration Never come across as selfish	Responsibility	It is down to me to protect/care/make things OK I make bad decisions My feelings are burdensome
I can't cope I should be dealing with this better I can't do what I need to do	Try your hardest to get what influence you have Never get your hopes up Never put yourself forward for things that you may fail at	Control/power	I don't have control I'm weak I am powerless/helpless I am a failure

Table 17: Prompts to explore motivations behind behaviours that may relate to threatening belief themes

Behaviours	Questions to explore	Potential related threatening belief theme/s
Constant busyness and difficulty resting or being	• What makes it uncomfortable not to be busy? • What does it mean to not be busy?	Safety Self-worth Control Responsibility
Avoidance of exertion or doing things that may be disrupted by symptoms	• What is the worst thing you fear if you get symptoms? • What implications would this have for you and your life?	Safety Self-worth
Prioritizing chores and obligations over pleasure	• What would it mean for you to prioritize pleasure for yourself each day? • What makes you feel most uncomfortable about this?	Self-worth Responsibility
Not talking about or disclosing health issues/difficulties when being hugely impacted by them	• What do you worry might happen if you shared your difficulties? • What's the worst thing about that for you?	Safety Self-worth Control
Trying every treatment regimen and supplement	• What does it mean to you if you don't try everything you can to improve things? • Does it mean something about you as a person? • What might it mean for your life?	Safety Control Responsibility

Constantly being on the watch for symptoms	• What do you worry might happen if you don't keep on high alert? • What do you think could be the repercussions of this?	Safety Control Responsibility
Never sharing difficult feelings or emotions	• What do you fear if you truly open up to someone? • What would you interpret this to mean about yourself or other people?	Control Safety Self-worth
Extensive planning and over-preparing for trips and activities	• What happens if you plan less? • What would that mean for your life?	Responsibility Safety
Being constantly distracted by the TV, social media and anything else so that there is no quiet time	• Are there things you worry would come up for you if you had less distraction? • What would be the effect of this on your life?	Safety Self-worth
Constantly questioning yourself, journaling and having long explorative conversations to better understand things	• What happens if you take action without working through all the options and potential repercussions? • Why do you think this feels so important to prevent or avoid?	Responsibility Control Self-worth

you might hold. Again, this is not a precise formula, but rather a good place to start investigating. Use Table 17 to see which (if any) behaviours you identify with. Use the next column to reflect on the questions and see if they help you identify which threatening belief themes may affect you. You can then use Table 16 to help you refine which beliefs may be most relevant for you.

Creating flexibility in beliefs

The more sense of personal effectiveness and meaning you have, the better your mental and physical health.[15] This has been shown across different patient populations including people recovering from cancer and with life-limiting illnesses.[16,17,18,19] Even before creating new beliefs, you can make more flexibility in old beliefs to allow for personal agency and meaning. I have adapted the concept of fixed versus growth mindset (popularized by Carol Dweck)[20] for application to broad health beliefs in Table 18. You may use it to cultivate flexibility for your own health beliefs where applicable.

Choosing your new beliefs

To reduce any brain resistance and make it feel emotionally safer to construct or adapt new beliefs, give yourself time to be intentional about what you want your new beliefs to be and what is realistic. Be gracious with yourself in the process of learning to believe them. You are, literally, physiologically rewiring your brain.

For one moment, set the book down and fold your arms now without thinking about it. Pick the book back up once you've done it. How was it to do that? Likely easy, without much of a second thought, for most of you. When you have your arms crossed it probably feels quite natural. Now, do it the other way round. Cross the opposite arm over the bottom arm. How is that? Chances are

Table 18: Adapting growth versus fixed mindset in application to global health beliefs

	Biomedical fixed mindset	Biopsychosocial growth mindset
Health challenge and adversity	Viewed as something to be fixed and sense of disempowerment to do much towards that	Viewed as an opportunity to learn, grow and overcome or adapt
Capability to navigate health and cope	Capabilities to cope with health difficulties are seen as fixed according to what they have been able to deal with in the past and unlikely to be changed in the face of further challenge and adversity	Capabilities are seen as something that can expand and be developed in response to challenges
Attitude towards effort to develop capabilities to navigate health and broader implications	Pointless and likely to fail as things are determined by biology and external medical professionals and systems. Pessimistic.	Essential to improve things and an opportunity to find ways to improve things and feel better. Optimistic.
Reaction to adversity, flare-ups and difficulties in the health journey	Viewed as evidence of lack of control and powerlessness.	Viewed as opportunities to reflect, regroup, and amend approach. Once less impacted by the emotional and physiological repercussion, the experience is consolidated as an opportunity to learn.

it is harder to do and feels odd. This is an embodiment of the internal process in your brain as you try to change beliefs. Your brain will want to default to the old pattern and feel uncomfortable in not being aligned. It will take more effort and calculation to remind yourself to do it the other way around. That is part of the process. Over time, it becomes more automated.

Picking new beliefs: a process

To keep things clear and feasible, focus on updating one old belief first rather than multiple beliefs at the same time.

1. Once you have identified your old belief to work on, using the guidance in previous sections write it down on the top of a sheet of paper. Underneath it, on one side of the page, write down all the ways this belief impacts you. Your feelings, your overall mood state, your interactions with people, your behaviour, your body and your health. Write as much as you can.
2. Now, next to that list, write down all the ways this belief has protected you and continues to protect you.
3. Reflect on the two lists. Is there an updated belief that can preserve some of the protection the old belief affords you, whilst reducing the negative impacts of it? Jot down your ideas. When coming up with alternative beliefs, you want to preserve some nuance but not make them too long. Use Table 19 if you need some inspiration. Create your own as feels resonant with your own experience.

Table 19: Old vs new beliefs

Old beliefs	New beliefs
I am weak	I have strength, weaknesses are not failures
I am not good enough	I have many qualities and can continue to grow
I am in danger	I can soothe myself and seek support
I am a burden	I am deserving of care
I'm trapped	I have choices
I am vulnerable	I can access safety
I don't matter	I have purpose/meaning

Embodying new beliefs

You can approach updating beliefs from two directions. The first is from the top-down (mind to body). Here you are working cognitively, intentionally appraising beliefs and creating alternatives. The practices so far in this chapter have been top-down strategies.

The second way to update beliefs is from the bottom-up. This is where you are embodying your alternative beliefs via your behaviour, shaping your beliefs by experience. When it is deemed safe, the new belief system will be readily adopted as it will feel preferable, both emotionally and physiologically. Bottom-up embodying of beliefs is truly fundamental for shifting beliefs. This involves:

- Identifying and planning actions that align with a new belief and can build up evidence for it
- Enacting those actions
- Logging experiences that are congruent with your new belief.

In Chapter 4, I introduced you to setting up behavioural experiments to help you move away from behaviours that feed vicious symptom spirals. You can use the same process to help create evidence for new beliefs and against old beliefs (page 161).

Having a journal or electronic document where you log evidence that supports the new belief helps your brain to 'learn' your new belief. Remember neurons that fire together, wire together? The more you are intentionally engaging with information that supports your updated belief, the more easily your brain can use these experiences and the belief itself as a frame of reference for understanding things. For example, if you were updating the belief 'I am insignificant' to 'I matter', you may intentionally reflect on moments where your assertiveness has paid off and when your partner has told you how much you mean to them. Then, when a friend appears disinterested when you share something, rather than your brain pinging back to 'I'm insignificant', it may be better able to retain that sense of mattering and contextualize accordingly.

Recognizing yourself as multidimensional

The pitfalls of dichotomous thinking and fixation on the self have been explored previously. When it comes to creating new beliefs about yourself, be mindful of the mind's tendency to reduce you to one thing and then elicit threat-detection processes that feed self-focus (again *not the same as* selfishness). This relates to tolerating uncertainty as mentioned earlier. Your brain may demand 100% proof that you matter (to use the example in the previous section). And this can make you feel *more* vulnerable, because in the absence of 100% certainty, your brain fears being proved wrong – you don't matter, after all. Aside from using the guidance for tolerating uncertainty (page 289) and attentional practices (page 164), you can powerfully counteract this threatened brain tendency by exploring your multidimensionality.

Exploring your multidimensionality

1. Write your name or sketch yourself out on a page (Figure 30). Around you, scribble down all the things you are, you do, you value and the connections and affiliations you have.
2. Spend some time reflecting on what aspects of you you'd like to explore more and brainstorm ideas about how you may do this. You don't have to action them all at once. Don't aim for that. Set yourself the intention of gently researching and exploring how you can cultivate these aspects of you more in a way that you'd like and that feels feasible.

My journey from 'I will never feel better' to 'things can be OK' was also a journey from 'I'm weak and pathetic' to 'I'm deserving of compassion'. In truth, there were many beliefs changing simultaneously as I navigated towards symptom remission and better mental health. The changing of these beliefs was by no means linear. It took repetition in the form of practising mindfulness in the moments where it felt good and the moments it felt like torture. It took putting myself out there (e.g. trying new things, changing habits, creating new connections) and feeling the intense anxiety of doing so, having to debrief and reconstruct things, when doing so was hard. It took lots of self-reflection and lots of social connection. All of this allowed me to weather the doubt that came in bucket loads at many points along the journey. As I persevered, more doors opened to help build these healthier beliefs further; from starting the health psychology master's, to engaging in research that widened my scope for what else was possible through cultivation of the mind–body connection. All of this paved the way for me to hold a strong, flexible and nuanced set of beliefs around myself, my health and my body.

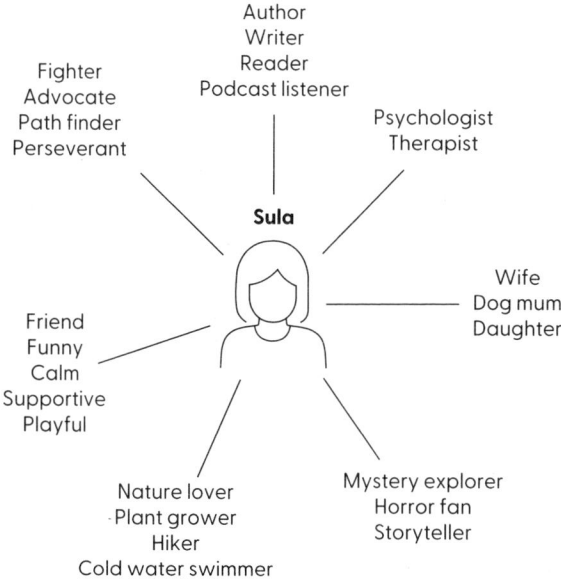

Figure 30: Example exploration of multidimensionality.

My journey became less about me trying to heal myself. When I had capacity, my focus shifted to how my experience could apply to others. Others like you.

This decentring of myself is one of the elements I credit most to my overall wellbeing. The times when I find myself feeling most vulnerable and distressed now are times when I feel utterly focussed on my problems. When there are things I cannot easily change, this can feel demoralizing. My clinic, my Instagram page, my writing, all keep me connected with my fellow humans. I cannot always shift my own reality, but I can find solace and beauty in helping others. Finding the balance between this and old people-pleasing beliefs of 'my needs aren't as important as others' is an ongoing journey. Remember this: you are a work in progress, and you always will be. I believe life is about the beauty of exploring, growing and developing. There is no satisfaction or meaning in being 'completed'. This makes it feel much safer to not be quite 'there yet'.

In this chapter you've become familiar with:

- What beliefs are and how they imprint physiologically with an effect on all aspects of life, including health
- How to harness neuroscience principles to develop and reinforce beliefs that create safety in mind and body
- How to embody new beliefs and embrace your multidimensionality.

There is a reason this chapter is towards the end of the book. Doing the work in the previous chapters, trying new things, getting new experiences, building metacognition, all helps the brain to be more open and malleable when it comes to this stage. It can feel safer to stray from old beliefs now that you've tried some things out for yourself gradually. As you come to the final chapter, take a moment to acknowledge yourself. What do you deserve credit for? What expectations have you perhaps been harbouring towards yourself to this point? What healing goals have you progressed and how do these experiences relate to beliefs you are exploring in this chapter? At the start of the chapter I wrote about how powerful your beliefs are in determining your experience of a moment and of future moments. My hope is that learning about how malleable your beliefs are has opened the potential for more freedom and empowerment now and in your future moments.

CHAPTER 9

A beautiful work in progress

The darkest moments of illness easily come back to me even now. Snapshots of grief and suffering. Waking up in a hospital bed after general anaesthetic, the tug of a catheter and crushing disappointment that the urethral camera had discovered no new answers on its journey into my inflamed bladder. Crumpling into myself moments later, on the toilet, after the catheter had been retracted. Immense pain traversing my genitals up to my stomach, painting a desolate view of my future. The black nights woken up abruptly by searing head pain, as though I'd been shot in the right temple. The voice at the other end of the phone during the one and only 111 call I'd made, telling me that there was nothing that could be done, as I clutched the cold wall, eyes tightly shut and wondering how I could continue with so much pain. Exposing my bare bum to a waiting room of outpatients and directed to the toilet by a nonplussed doctor after another invasive diagnostic test caused my bladder to misfire. The agony after a bike ride on holiday, throwing me into mental spirals.

To this day, when I allow myself to go back there, I can feel the tug in my heart, the semblance of tension in my pelvis and the tightening of my jaw.

I don't pity past Sula. I have admiration for her. I recognize how alone she often was at her most vulnerable and how she still found ways to wedge open gaps of hope and run with them when she could. To remember the suffering is to marvel at the perseverance. I have infinite love for her and how much her actions led me to where I am now. In a body that I can care for and that works with me to the best of its capacity.

My story is one of complete symptom remission, which is an amazing privilege. One that is not possible for everyone, depending on your health, capacity, environment and any of the many other biopsychosocial influencers of health. Although symptom remission is something I'm endlessly grateful for and was indeed my only aim at the outset, my conceptualization of 'getting better' evolved as I navigated the journey.

What started as 'will I *ever* get better?' gave way to '*when* will I get better?' as I improved my physical and emotional experience through mindfulness, medication, social connection, emotional processing and more. Here, still, my emphasis was on physical remission. As symptoms receded, the crisis of being unwell receded enough for me to start wondering 'who am I now that I'm getting better?' This can be a confronting question. The experience of breaking down after trying to make friends in my new city, as described in Chapter 5, gives some indication of how confronting it was for me. Much may have changed in the time you have been dealing with crisis: friendships, relationships, work, sense of self and more. The world around you may feel as changed as you are. As you navigate this and find your new normal, the questions don't stop. Your brain may instead look for '*what* do I want to be better now?' As a human, finding ways to enhance your experience is baked into your biology. It's a biological predisposition that can be wielded for growth and life satisfaction or for impatience and disharmony, depending on how it's channelled.

This chapter will guide you to nurture the evolving conceptualization of 'getting better' as you reach different stages in your healing journey. I'll provide you with principles to tether yourself in the present safely, even when things are hard, while maintaining motivation for bettering the open road ahead. Together we'll acknowledge the importance of endings, what they represent and how they feel.

You are not your illness or disability

When illness starts or worsens to the point that it takes up all the available space in your life, and who you are or what you want is squeezed out to the sidelines, it can be hard to re-emerge when symptoms are not *as* all-consuming, without the right support and guidance. When symptoms have created long-term disruption, or they are a permanent fixture, it can feel like there is no 're-emerging'. The more room your illness or difficulties take up and the less support and acceptance you get from others, the less room there is for *you*.

Working with people across a spectrum of physical symptoms (e.g. fatigue, bowel and bladder issues, pain, brain fog) and severity of symptoms, I have seen how even in the context of terminal illness or high symptom complexity, there is a way for 'self' and illness to co-exist peacefully. Research shows that people who find this blend between their illness and their sense of self tend to feel better physically and emotionally while retaining better physical function than those who either strongly reject their illness or feel consumed by it.[1]

The term researchers have coined for feeling consumed by illness is 'engulfment'. Your symptoms and related challenges have taken over your vision of yourself so that it feels like your illness is who you are. This can feel protective because it ensures you tend to your health, when no one else seems to prioritize that, and it can make you part of a community of others who have the same challenges as you.

As we've considered, the sense of connection and being part of something *is* important. The problem with engulfment is that it can be hard to find the traces of you outside the illness and this blending reduces your perception of control or influence. Mild symptoms may seem automatically indicative of a flare-up round the corner, necessitating an immediate countermeasure. For example, feeling drowsy in the afternoon after lunch may be interpreted as a sinister symptom of your condition that requires you to cancel plans and rest. In contrast, when there is more separation between your identity and illness, there may be room to imagine that the drowsiness is a result of the natural afternoon slump after eating, with the possibility of passing as the day goes on. You can then take more moderate steps like cutting plans slightly shorter. In Chapter 4, we explored how thoughts about symptoms, emotional reactions and ensuing responses can significantly affect the trajectory of symptoms and longer-term health outcomes. Engulfment creates more negative symptom spirals, worsening health and mental health outcomes.[2]

Working out how to separate yourself from your illness when it is all-consuming, maybe especially so during specific parts of your health journey, is difficult. The chapters in this book have included two elements in parallel: 1) information and strategies focussed specifically on improving symptom experience, and 2) information and strategies focussed on nurturing you and your sense of self. Developing both together helps you balance illness and sense of self. Figure 31 shows the distinction between being engulfed by illness, attempting to reject it entirely and accepting it. We'll consider acceptance more centrally in later parts of this chapter.

I don't know who I am any more

Working with people who have multiple health diagnoses, spanning years (even decades), who have navigated the many rungs of the healthcare system and may have found themselves ejected

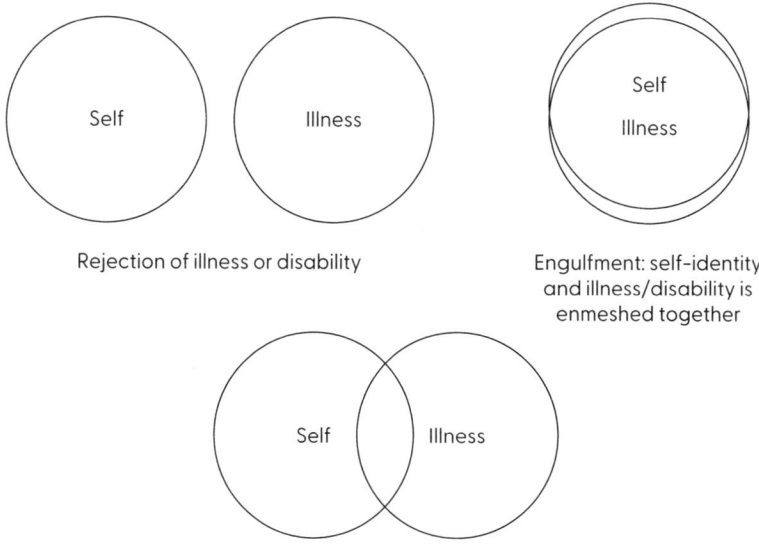

Figure 31: Depiction of ways that your sense of self and illness can exist.

again after years of symptoms and procedures, I often hear this sentiment: 'I miss who I used to be.' There have been so many health crises, so much focus on basic survival, that the question of 'who are you and what do you want?' will have long-since felt superfluous. *I have no option to get what I want even if I knew?!*

The natural order of things in your mind may be something like 'get better, *then* consider the bigger life questions'. While this is intuitive, it can also obscure opportunities for healing along the way. It is best not to suspend exploration of who you are and your sense of meaning until you are 'better' because you lose opportunities for healing and for counterbalancing allostatic load.

To find the sweet spot between pragmatism and honouring your deeper needs, the question of who you are can be explored in different ways at different phases of your journey:[3]

- **Crisis:** You are in the midst of uncertainty and disruption
- **Coping:** You are attempting different things to cope and find some kind of balance
- **Adaptation:** You have found ways to cope and engage with life that work for you.

The first phase of the health journey is one of crisis and disruption, grappling with physical and emotional disruption to life as you know it. While the question of who you are isn't a priority, you continue to embody who you are. It's there in how you relate to your experience, how you process, how you manage your feelings. Naturally all these processes can be hugely impeded by biological threat processes, that fuel negative symptom spirals.

'Coping' comes after crisis. You explore (perhaps with urgency) what you can do to help yourself and what support is out there. It involves experimentation and analysis. It can be full of hope, followed by disappointment as things that felt sure to help don't seem to bring the results you'd hoped for. This can push you back into crisis mode. Just as you have before, you can again get yourself back into coping. There can be a bit of back and forth between crisis and coping, but eventually all of that back and forth like a pendulum can swing you into the adaptation phase.

The adaptation phase is characterized by stability and balance. You have found ways to integrate illness/disability into life so that you can have a sense of meaning, pleasure and connection. This involves adapting around your condition. Even with full remission, the adaptation phase means working with your body in a way that continues to respect its limits and need for nurturing.

Considering the question of who you want to be while in the coping phase can propel you into the adaptation phase quicker and more smoothly. Adaptation becomes much harder without considering this because *you* and what matters to *you* is absent from your coping strategies. It has become all about symptom remediation. Everything that you used to enjoy, your habits, your

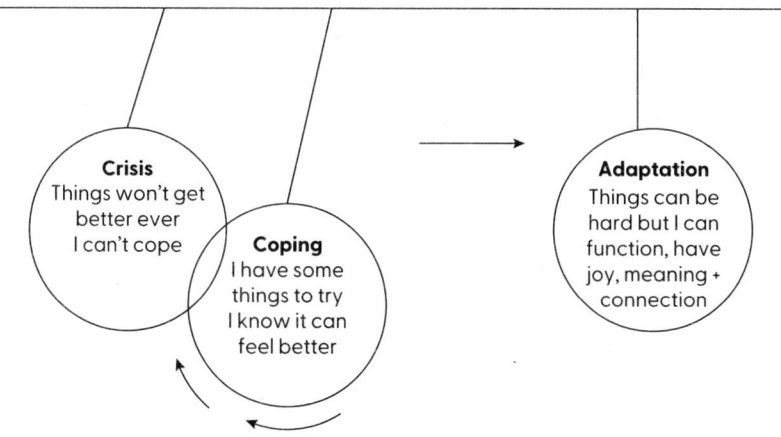

Figure 32: Illustration of how you may swing back and forth between coping and crisis before reaching the adaptation phase.

goals, may have been entirely washed away with the tide of illness. The brain and broader biology defaults to threat mode, which inhibits more integrated long-term thriving in the adaptation phase.

Finding yourself

If you can find yourself during suffering, you can enhance yourself in health. As true as this is, let's set some expectations. In times of crisis or extreme overwhelm, exploring who you are can add to the overwhelm. Give yourself licence to come back to this when you have the bandwidth. If you feel you are in a place with enough headspace to be explorative, to appraise your coping in the wider view of your life, then it may be an opportune time to do the following exercise. This exercise is one taken from acceptance and commitment therapy (ACT). As Russ Harris, a renowned trainer of ACT, said on one of his trainings I joined, ACT has a 'branding problem'. We may equate acceptance with resignation: the giving in to things staying the same and remaining powerless.

Far from that, acceptance is a reclamation of resources. Resources that are otherwise expended on fighting against things that you have limited power to change. Acceptance is a willingness to turn towards difficult things and working *with* them rather than against them. This involves openness, curiosity and willingness. It also requires an alternative tether for you to reorient yourself towards, away from the single focus of wanting things to be different. This is where the exercise comes in.

The practice: setting your values to find yourself

The purpose of this practice is to connect with the things that are important to you in life. Your threat-focussed brain may find it hard to quantify this without considering your present difficulties. It will be concerned with measuring up how practically you can enact things that are important to you, while you are experiencing what you are currently experiencing. As best you can, try to suspend reality. Working out the practicalities comes later down the line. Your task for this practice is to simply imagine and explore what intuitively comes up for you.

You may find it helpful to do this practice several times and come back to it as you journal, reflect further and explore with trusted others. This may be the first time you are consciously quantifying what you value in life, and it is an important moment. You can use the audio for this or the prompts below.*

Picture yourself at an advanced age and being at peace with this, having lived a fulfilling life. You are celebrating your birthday and someone gives a speech about you. Consider what you would like to hear them say about you and how you showed up across these aspects of life:

---

* Audio link available at www.healthpsychologist.co.uk/itsallinyourbody

- Private leisure time
- As a family member
- As a friend
- Spiritually or self-transcendence.

You can use Table 20 to help you identify core values that guide each area of your life.

As you describe the values, try to explore why the values are important to you and how they can feature in these areas of your life. Multiple values may resonate. Select the values that feel most poignant.

Three main concerns can come up in this practice:

- Being old and the losses associated with that (parents or loved ones no longer there, the passage of time, a sense of waste of younger years)
- The absence of sufficient connection or support (what if no one will be there?)
- How far values feel from life now.

These become barriers to connecting with your values. If this happens to you as you attempt this exercise, you may like to process some of those difficult feelings first by using the guidance from Chapter 5. Come back to this practice with the intention of connecting with these values and how they can give you a sense of meaning and fulfilment even if that is currently minimal.

Research that shows that identifying and acting in accordance with your values and sense of purpose protects you from burnout, improving your mood and overall wellbeing.[4] It also has major health benefits, with some studies showing links between your length of life and your sense of purpose.[5]

Table 20: List of values		
Altruism	Ethics	Leadership
Accomplishment	Fairness	Love
Active	Faith	Loyalty
Adventure	Flexibility	Meaning
Ambition	Freedom	Nature
Authenticity	Fulfilment	Nurturing
Awareness	Fun	Openness
Balance	Generosity	Optimism
Belonging	Geniality	Patience
Braveness	Grace	Peace
Caring	Gratitude	Perseverance
Collaboration	Growth	Power
Commitment	Harmony	Resourcefulness
Compassion	Honesty	Respect
Connection	Humility	Safety
Contentment	Humour	Self-compassion
Courage	Independence	Self-expression
Creativity	Integrity	Serenity
Curiosity	Intuition	Spirituality
Dedication	Joy	Trusting
Determination	Justice	Trustworthy
Diligence	Kindness	Understanding
Divinity	Knowledge gatherer	Uniting
Equality	Knowledge sharer	Wisdom

Penny's story

I've already talked a bit about how values offer an alternative to fighting against things you have no control over, by orienting you towards things that can better serve you. One of my clients, Penny, had multiple sclerosis (MS) and had been told that it was progressive. Her symptoms were predicted to worsen, and she would lose more physical functioning. She often felt full of fear about what this would look like. This fear would send her into hours of researching worst-case scenarios and obscure treatments that seemed hopeless. She was mainly housebound due to her mobility, and she would ruminate on what she had already lost, falling into despair when the fear of what was to come spiralled again. Penny knew none of this helped her, but she felt helpless to stop it.

When she started connecting with her values, she remembered how creative she had been and was still. The creativity had been forgotten along the way. When she reconnected with it, a long-dormant part of her was instantly rekindled. Like it had just been waiting for her to turn her attention back to it. She had a flurry of ideas of how she may create art, even with limited dexterity. Not just that, she considered with excitement how she could start consuming art again, listening to certain radio shows and even in her time spent watching the garden. She could apply her artist's eye whilst listening to music. I was amazed at how easily her creativity reignited, with what seemed like the mere mention of something that had been important to her.

The next time I came to see her she had beautiful art to show me. 'Yes, I'm still depressed,' she smiled at me, 'but it's been lovely to get back into this.' She told me how she had plans to bestow some of her creations to people who meant something to her. There was a vibrancy to her, and to her discussion of this, that I'd not seen before. This vibrancy sustained and grew across the sessions we had together.

As you begin to feel more alignment with your purpose and connected with your authentic self, you are less likely to rely on things that deplete you physiologically (e.g. fatty diet, quick dopamine fixes from digital overstimulation, etc.) and you are more likely to have a physiological buffer against the negative impacts of stress. People with a high sense of enacted purpose have less inflammation,[6] enhanced cellular immunity[7] and healthier heart rate variability.[8] Your body rewards you for honouring yourself because it feels safe and replenished when you do so.

You are multidimensional

In Chapter 8, we saw how negative beliefs about yourself can mean that your sense of worth is dictated by a tunnel-visioned set of criteria that you can only achieve or fail at. Needing to be productive or likeable or accomplished can overshadow the other rich aspects of you, minimizing their importance when the reality is that you are not one thing, but many. You have different roles, different ways to express yourself, different moods and different seasons of life. Embracing the different dimensions of you allows your life to be colourful and abundant even in the face of adversity. The problem is that you are often dragged back by your brain (and society) into dichotomous appraisals of yourself (e.g. failing, weak).

Having become acquainted with your values, the next invitation is to start using them to lean into your multidimensionality and update old rigid beliefs. When I was in the early stages of recovering from my bladder issues, I did not feel able to go to the gym because it always seemed to cause a flare of my symptoms. At that time, I was trying to apply for the master's programme, do my full-time job and navigate other elements of health that were still uncertain. Prior to getting ill, I'd gone to the gym at least three times a week for three years or so. It was how I connected with my body, felt good about myself and it shaped how I saw myself as a 'fit' person.

If old negative belief systems had been running the show, I may have felt like I was failing, feeling anxious about what stepping back from the gym would mean for my appearance, for my health and anything else related to that. These self-perceptions could so easily have undermined all my efforts in other areas of life. Instead, I was able to embrace the spectrum of values I had, recognizing that many of them were being nurtured. Educationally, I was pursuing further knowledge for self-growth and to contribute to the greater good, with hopes to conduct research that would help others. I was connecting with my friends more and I was nurturing and being nurtured in my relationships. I was caring for my body in alternative ways that were more suited to my physical circumstances. Looking at myself and my experience in this way was so much more reflective of reality and so much more nourishing. It meant that guilt or anxiety about not going to the gym was short-lived and tolerable.

As you learn to update old, inaccurate, reductive beliefs, you will find it easier to simultaneously turn towards your values to guide you more flexibly. This supports the creation and reinforcement of new neural pathways, allowing old ones to fall away. Each time you notice old beliefs in action, and you intentionally turn towards your values for guidance, you are reinforcing these healthier, more sustaining neural pathways.

The next exercise helps you to do this by prioritizing which values you want to intentionally nurture and cultivate more at this time in your life. Remember, you will go through different phases in recovery and different seasons of life. You can reuse this practice when it feels like your priorities need to shift.

The practice

Organize the values you identified as important to you in the previous practice, using Table 21.*

1. Rate how important each value is to you to embody right now in this phase of your life on a scale of 0–10, where 0 is neutral rather than unimportant, and 10 is the most important that they could be.
2. Rate how aligned (how much you enact or embody) you feel with each value in each area of life, where 0 is not aligned at all,

---

* A blank template is available at www.healthpsychologist.co.uk/itsallinyourbody

and 10 is the most aligned you could be. Try not to judge yourself whatever the rating. Life is hard, health issues, burnout and mood states naturally move you away from your values. This is why you are doing this exercise – give yourself credit for that.

3. Now you have your importance versus alignment ratings, you can prioritize which areas rate highest on importance and lowest on alignment. If there are many areas, pick three, maximum, to focus on.

In Table 21, the underlined importance and alignment ratings indicate good choices to focus on because the importance is high, but the alignment is lower. To further filter down from the 6 underlined, you could focus on one area of life, such as friendship. Another option is to focus on one value from each area of life where the alignment is lower. Working on values across different areas of life can complement each other simultaneously. Prioritize according to what resonates with you and what feels feasible.

From those areas you've identified that don't feel aligned with your values, use the prompts below to explore:

- What has made it hard to connect with your values in this area?
- What has it felt like to feel disconnected from your values in this area?
- What would it mean to you, to reconnect with this value in this area of life?
- What could that look like? What sorts of things would you be doing or no longer doing?
- Are there resources that you need to help to realign yourself with this value? List them even if they don't feel accessible resources right now.
- What is one small action you can make consistently to better connect you to your value/s in particular areas of your life?

Table 21: Identifying values and rating importance and alignment			
Area of life	Value	Importance	Alignment
Free time for leisure, fun, hobbies	E.g. To be playful	8	7
Family	E.g. Caring Knowledge sharer	9 6	9 7
Friendships	E.g. Authentic Fair Open Fun	9 8 9 8	4 10 9 7
Intimate relationships	E.g. Fun Nurturing Trustworthy	8 9 10	8 9 10
Spirituality/ transcendence	E.g. Nature lover Creative	8 8	6 5
Profession/ education	E.g. Dedicated Perseverant Knowledge gatherer	8 7 9	10 10 10
Health and wellbeing	E.g. Nurturing of my body Self-compassionate Active	10 9 8	7 4 7

Post-traumatic growth

Being confronted by your body's vulnerabilities and experiencing changes in mood that feel out of your control can be traumatic. As we've seen, trauma changes how your brain processes events, keeping it stuck at the point/s of extreme threat and lack of safety. This is why it is so important to work with your biology as you try and help yourself psychologically and practically navigate challenges of burnout and illness. As you do so, things start to feel less threatening, you begin to feel more empowered and that creates space for something else: post-traumatic growth.

Post-traumatic growth is a concept originating in the 1990s and defined as 'positive psychological changes experienced as a result of the struggle with trauma or highly challenging situations'.[9] Here are some of the ways that it shows up:

- Feeling more appreciative and connected to oneself
- Feeling a greater purpose and able to action it
- Being able to appreciate the small pleasures and wins
- Having compassion and empathy for fellow humans
- Being invested in nurturing oneself and others
- Kinship with similarly affected groups
- New possibilities opening from a shift in life path
- Feeling more confident in your own personal strength.

I've worked with many people who were entrenched on a particular life course that felt completely jeopardized by illness. They came to me with extreme depression, despairing as they grappled with the difficulties of getting back to their envisioned life path. Only to find that once they'd worked through the grief and reconnected with their body, they no longer desired this path. CEOs have chosen to step back from huge deals in favour of philanthropic pursuits; hungry young executives have decided to pursue careers without lavish bonuses but with a better work-life balance; self-subjugating women mistreated in hostile social circles have realized they deserve friendships that can truly offer a sense of belonging. Whether it is seeing their old life pursuits as unfulfilling or identifying old patterns as misguided and unsustainable, the sense of having *really* discovered oneself in amongst the rubble is beautiful.

What I've observed about post-traumatic growth is that once you have it, you have it for life. No matter what comes, there is something steely and comforting within you that steadies you in stormy times. It can go a little quiet in extreme overwhelm, but it always reappears, ready to help you navigate.

What aids post-traumatic growth?

One key factor is timing. If you are still experiencing trauma or are in the crisis phase of health issues, much-needed defences (physical, psychological and social) will keep active. You may be growing from these experiences, but you must focus on surviving them. Equally, when in these experiences, feeling positively about any of it may be impossible or even unhelpful. I certainly could not have found any convincing benefits when festering in my bed after the eleventh excruciating trip to the toilet and nor would I expect myself to in that situation. Going back to the stages of the health journey, during the crisis and coping stages, you are cultivating the ingredients that can transform into post-traumatic growth in the adaptation phase.[10]

During the coping stage, the things that shift you towards post-traumatic growth are all the things we have explored in the pages of this book, right up to this chapter. Research has highlighted elements that have the strongest link with post-traumatic growth:[11]

- **Valued action**. Taking affirmative value-aligned action towards your goals as explored in this chapter is a big part of post-traumatic growth.
- **Cognitive processing**. Being able to acknowledge thoughts that are painful and scary and to intentionally explore how you feel about yourself (Chapter 8).
- **Social support**. Feeling connected with people who understand and accept you, and having a broader sense of belonging facilitates post-traumatic growth as well as bodily homeostasis (Chapter 7).
- **Feeling positive or optimistic**. Being able to embrace the full spectrum of emotions aids your ability to connect with a

sense of hope and the ability to savour comfort, joy and pleasure (Chapter 5).

Sidestepping toxic positivity

Post-traumatic growth is something that tends to grow organically from engaging in the practices included in this book. It is not something I'd suggest you aim for directly because it can lead you astray and into the realms of emotional suppression and over-responsibility. You can recognize this happening when you don't allow yourself to acknowledge or spend time with difficulties, because 'you should be over it' or 'you should be grateful because now . . .' or any self-talk that starts with 'at least' and ends with a blocking of difficult feelings.

The key to sidestepping toxic positivity is making space for multiple realities and experiences together. It can still feel hard some days, and, at the same time, you are able to appreciate the comforts you have now. You can be grateful for all that you've learnt whilst still mourning what you used to have.

Your next steps

One of my former PhD supervisors invited me and a group of my fellow students for dinner, to mark the ending of our PhDs. Some of us had moved institutions, others had stayed on but changed into post-doctoral roles, others were going on to do further training. We sat looking towards our supervisor at the head of her ample table, with flutes of champagne, as she told us that an old supervisor of hers had once said that it was important to acknowledge endings. The minute she said it I had an instant visceral reaction I didn't fully understand in that moment. She went on to acknowledge the collective and individual endings. The visceral reaction crystallized into a feeling of grief that felt familiar. Things were about to change. My community was once again about to disperse.

We can shy away from this, but that leaves us partially blinded. Endings and change are an inevitability of life and the more we can embrace them, extract the beauty and go forth with intention, aligned with our values, the more fulfilled we can feel as we journey through life.

As you come to the final pages of this book, identify what it is that you feel. At the end of therapy, you may imagine that people skip off feeling unburdened and 'cured', but that's not quite how it goes. *I* am not the active ingredient of their therapy, I am merely the facilitator. I've witnessed incredible changes: going from celibacy because of pelvic pain or bladder infections, to birthing healthy babies; going from being housebound to reclaiming independence, leaving the house daily, socializing freely and even resuming studies. For some the physicality of conditions could not change, but the internal world went from bleak and hopeless to meaningful and empowered. No matter the transformation, there remains a level of healthy trepidation at the end of therapy. This is because my clients recognize from the work they have already done that the process will be an ongoing one that takes maintenance.

That maintenance will evolve as you do.

You can use the guidance below to help you navigate your onwards journey and extract the maximum benefit from this book.

- **Review your goals.** In the Introduction, you were guided to create two types of goals: outcome goals and process goals. As you have moved through the book, you may have refined these process goals already as you gained clarity on what processes needed targeting to move you towards your outcome goal(s).

    Now that you have more knowledge and perhaps experience, it is the perfect time to review these goals. If you have a brain that is prone to telling you off for not having achieved your goals completely, let me help you out. At the beginning of the book, you weren't in the best position to create your goals because you didn't know what you know now. But you had to start somewhere and orient your journey through this book. Think about your initial goal-setting like the first draft of a book. I don't mind telling you that I drafted my proposal for this very book years before I finished the final proposal. It took many drafts and now this final manuscript is quite removed from the initial draft proposal, but you know what? Without that first proposal, neither you nor I would be here at this sentence.

See if you now want to update your goals. Note where you have made changes if you have, however small, and curiously explore how this feels and what this means to you. It is important to acknowledge your micro-wins on a psychological and physiological level because this is rewarding for your brain and motivates you to keep going (progress principle). It also makes you feel more accomplished and safer in your body.

- **Map the chapters to your goals.** Now that you have updated your goals, map out which process goals can be supported by which chapters in this book. Plan out how you will use these chapters and the suggested exercises, as well as any other resources you have,* to move towards your goals over the next one to two months. This part can be broad and messy as you look at the various strands you want to work on.
- **Prioritize your focus for the next one to two months.** If you have lots of goals that relate to lots of different sections of this book, cross-reference your goals against the values exercise you have done in this chapter. Which goals best overlap with

---

* Additional resources and signposting available at www.healthpsychologist.co.uk/itsallinyourbody

the valued areas you have prioritized? Use this to guide you to pick the areas you want to prioritize over the next one to two months. Refine things further, by creating clear intentions related to these value-informed goals, that you can implement each week (e.g. I will reach out to a friend to chat at least once a week, I will check in with my body using the nervous system barometer daily, I will spot areas I find it hard to assert myself and practise assertive communication).

As part of this process, identify the daily micro-habits that can keep you aligned with these goals (e.g. savouring, noticing your feelings, spotting thoughts, nurturing your body in a specific way like keeping hydrated or regular bedtime).

- **Pick a time to reflect.** I often encourage clients of mine to pick a 'self-therapy' appointment with themselves regularly. This might be weekly, fortnightly or monthly, but it is scheduled in. The time is spent checking in on goals, noting where you've drifted from your intentions, reflecting on the triumphs and challenges and problem-solving. I've created some prompts for your self-therapy check-ins:

  - What goals did you set out to work on?
  - What progress have you made (however small)?
  - How does this feel? What difference has this made to you (however small)?
  - What are the challenges you've faced in working towards these goals?
  - What can help with these challenges?
  - What support could you do with and what options are there for finding this support?

A powerful exercise I sometimes incorporate into the end of therapy is writing a letter to yourself. The idea is that you write this letter to help the you in three months' time, for whom all of this isn't quite so fresh, who may be veering off from goals or finding things hard again. As you write this letter, you want to include all the things that can help ground and inspire the future you, who could do with the reminder. What do you want them to know, having read this book, that captures how you feel now?

Use these prompts to help guide your letter to yourself:

- What has stood out to you from reading this book? What resonated and why?
- What felt hard to hear and what was comforting?
- What things feel important but unresolved or unclear?
- How has this book helped you better understand yourself and your resolve to look after you and perhaps others too?
- What tools, strategies or sentiments could be particularly helpful for future you to remember?

Write the letter and save it somewhere. You can do this pen to paper or electronically. Wherever you save it, schedule a reminder or email to yourself to tell you to check it out in three months.

I'm still not done

When I worked in the NHS, it was standard for patients to only receive six to twelve sessions of therapy, no matter how complex their physical or psychological presentations were. That meant that someone who was being denied benefits, whilst unable to work, with four chronic conditions and long-term depression, was expected to 'get better' in the same time frame as someone who had no environmental adversity, one specific goal for therapy and no additional physical comorbidities. While I truly believe that some therapeutic provision (delivered appropriately in the time frame) is better than none, I also feel that time-limited therapy can misrepresent healing journeys as short and linear. It can shape expectations that you should heal all in one go – never to return to therapy. Returning to therapy from this perspective can feel a lot like failing.

When I moved to private practice, where there were no strict cut-offs, I had the privilege of joining people for much longer on their healing journeys. I was able to see the twists and turns and periods where it felt like nothing had changed, only for things to shift and all their prior hard work to come good. Many of my clients have worked with multiple therapists before me. Those experiences of therapy have often contributed to their progress in therapy with me. They created foundations that we could build on, making it possible to reach the goals we set for therapy this time round.

You may have made some definitive goals using this book, that you are now working towards. Don't make the mistake of downing tools once you reach those goals. Healing takes maintenance and intentionality. I've been in remission from bladder symptoms for over a decade at the point of writing this book, and I am still learning about myself and my bladder. The world around me changes, my body responds, and I notice changes within myself. None of us are static. We are hurtling through space and time, gradually aging and encountering different experiences. Although it is natural to resist change and the threats it can pose, cultivating curiosity and being open to what else you can discover across the different seasons of life brings safety and ease, even in the most uncertain of times. You've got time to explore, to go in different directions and to repeat yourself. All of this is integral to growth and healing. Challenge fuels change.

My story is about so much more than symptom remission. It is about the depth of despair I felt that shaped my pursuit of preventing those experiences for others. It is about the discovery of truly sustaining friendship, partnership and love and the beauty and wholeness this brings to the world. It is about discovering comfort and safety in my own authenticity, divorced from culturally informed metrics that make me feel hollow. It is about being at peace with what I can't know, open to what I don't know and welcoming of new wisdom.

As I come to the close of writing this final passage, there are many parallels to moments where I was at my most ill. Wrapped in a knitted cardigan, buried under a blanket with an array of water bottles and cups around me, I am once again looking bedraggled with greasy hair and a blank stare. Only this time, the quilt is for comfort not a sense of protection from the outside world. Back then I would fearfully try and flood my bladder to prevent my urine from burning, meaning I was never without water. Now, the cups are simply evidence of my commitment to adequately hydrate and nourish my body. Once, the bedraggled appearance and blank stare was because I'd given up. This time, they result from my determination to hand in a manuscript that may prevent others feeling as I did then.

I conjure up young, scared Sula once more now. Taking in her silent dejection as she lies alone in the dark, buried under her quilt, barely audible TV casting blue light on her face. Her mind is blank.

I tell her now:

Sula, your suffering is real and raw and I'm so sorry that you feel it. Your body is screaming, and you can't understand that now, but you will. You'll realize how your body isn't betraying you but pleading for things you don't yet recognize you need. But you will. Don't trouble yourself with the pressures of knowing everything. That is too much of a burden for you. Right now, you may feel alone but know that you are not. Your journey to fully discover this will not be straightforward but there will be much beauty to it, if you can only look for it. I promise that as you do, you'll discover more beauty and meaning than you can ever imagine right now.

Wherever *you* are in your journey, I hope you are finding a way to work with yourself; with your mind and with your body, engendering a sense of trust between the two so that you can have trust in yourself. That by recognizing the biopsychosocial nature of health (and life in general), you are recognizing that you have agency for change but no blame to claim. Your healing is not all on you. I hope that this book can be a comforting companion as you navigate seasons of life you've yet to explore, with an open heart to connection and community that can hold you in your times of vulnerability. You are not on your own.

I hope that knowing there is much of your story yet to come will give you a sense of hope because you are a beautiful work in progress.

Acknowledgements

In testament to the idea that our social world shapes us, I owe deep thanks to the many people whose support and influence helped bring this book into being. My husband, Matthew, who in the early stages of symptom remission, talked me into believing that I could go back to university to do a master's in health psychology. I believe you profoundly changed my life as you *saw* me and nurtured me in sickness and in health. Your words of encouragement, oxytocin hugs, jokes and matchas have sustained me throughout this writing process and more.

I'm grateful to my mum, Susan, the only reader of my early drafts, fellow writer and valuable sounding board as well as cheerleader. I still grin as I remember your scream of excitement when you heard I was writing a book. Thank you to my dad, Eric. You have always supported my love of learning, books and my journey through sickness and to mindfulness. Sue, without your words of wisdom about the processes of pain, perhaps none of this would be so. Thank you for giving me transformative hope and insight.

A special credit to my editors at Macmillan. Cara Waudby-Tolley, your sensitive and skilful edits have shaped the book to where it is today and are truly valued. I have often felt physically warmed by your lovely comments and insights. Lizzy Gray, thank you for seeing the vision for this book, significantly guiding my writing in early drafts and assembling a great team.

My agents, Lauren Gardner and Callen Martin, your industry expertise, debriefs, organization and encouragement have made the process of writing my first book nothing but exciting and comfortable. Thank you. I must also thank the early champions of the book who generously wrote their support for the concept before a single word was written: Dr Frances Ryan, Clare Bourne, Sophie Medlin, Nicole Vignola, Roisin Dervish Okane and Dr Hazel Wallace.

I have had so many mentors along the way, including my PhD supervisors Trudie, Rona and Kim, whose expertise, knowledge and pastoral care helped me develop personally as well as professionally. I'll always remember the King's College London Health Psychology Department fondly – to the entire department – you know who you are, thank you for the years of academic stimulation and collegiate fun.

To the 'Health Psych Girls', Alicia, Alice, Susan, Whitney and Zoe – how amazing that I could cite my friends' research in this book. From London Bridge to Scotland, you guys embody 'social safety' and were in my mind as I wrote Chapter 7.

I must also thank Joe and Leroy, our talks on walks about the world, therapy and relationships significantly shaped this book. Hannah Poulter, my fellow university-drop-out-cum-psychology-student-enroller – as I let you know how much your fierce friendship has meant to me, I picture us in our onesies as students revising and chanting study authors' names 'Abyanker ...'

I'm grateful to all those who have trusted me to facilitate a part of their journey in therapy. Your courage, openness and insights continue to inspire me. A special thank you also to the beautiful members of the Body Mind Connect community, whose willingness to connect and share, despite having experienced many social threats, is truly moving.

Lastly, thank you to the incredible researchers, clinicians and writers whose work I have cited, dedicated to improving things for their fellow humans.

Index

Note: page numbers in **bold** refer to diagrams, page numbers in *italics* refer to information contained in tables.

acceptance 133, 182–3, 207, 306, 309–10
acceptance and commitment therapy (ACT) 211, 309
acetylcholine 44, 199
aches 52–3, 81, 226
achievement focus 155, 230
acne 98
action 35
  collective *262*
  compassionate 260
  valued 319
adaptation phase 308–9, **309**
adenomyosis 94, 234
adenosine 139–40
adjustment phase 11
adrenaline 42–4, 123, 152, 236
adversity 12, 13, 17, 261, 264, 267, 283, 285, *296*, 314
advice, unsolicited 13
affirmational support **256**
agency 17, 66, 73, 239, 248, 277–8, 282, 295, 327
aggression 238, 246–8, *247*, 252
aging 15, 239–45

alcohol consumption 137, 236, 251
alexithymia 177
alignment 315–16, *317*
allergies 69, 87, 97
allostatic load (chronic stress) 51–2, 54, 56–7, 62–3, 76, 109, 145–6, 179, 188, 198, 239, 244, 254, 285, **285**, 307
alopecia 98
altriusm *262*
American Psychological Association (APA) 261
amygdala 16, 20, 47, 49, 71, 73–4, 110, 120–1, 216, 226, 236
  amygdala hijack 49, 113, 162, 171
Ancient Greeks 233–4
Angelou, Maya 239
anger 4, 7, 8, 74–5, 99–100, 124, 166, 171, 193–4, 210
anterior cingulate cortex (ACC) 20, 73–4, 171, 175, 178, 199, 207, 226
anterior insula 171, 175, 178, 207, 220
anti-inflammatories, natural 44

anxiety 3, 21, 70–2, 94, 96, 98, 109, 120, 127, 164, 169, 171, 173, 185–6, 265
  and assertiveness 248
  bodily experience of 175, 176
  and decentring 257
  and distraction 188
  and expressive writing 189–90
  and hypervigilance 162
  and mindfulness 208
  and misdiagnosis of heart attack in women 234
  and multidimensionality 300, 314, 315
  and nervous system activation 143
  of over-achievers 290
  and physical symptoms 244
  and safety behaviours 121–2
  and sleep 79
  social 56, 58, 165, 257
  spirals of 115
  and uncertainty 289
anxiety disorders 129
aphantasia 221
arthritis 62, 85, 239
assertiveness 246–68, *247*, 252
attachment 14–15, 254–5, *284*, 285
attention 82–3, 187, 191, 198–200, **199**, 202–3, 205–6, 283–5, 299
attention deficit hyperactivity disorder (ADHD) 152, 162, 242, *243*, 245
attentional habits 162–5
attentional spotlight 163–5, 257
authenticity 313, 326
autism 162, 177, 242, *243*, 245
autoimmunity 83–6, 97, 207–8, 227, 229

autonomic nervous system (ANS) 41–2, 44–6, 71, 75, 82, 91, 92, 97, 124, 141–4, 146, 182, 199, 211, 236
  activated state 142–4, **142**, **143**, *144*
  balanced state 142–4, **142**, **143**, *144*
  deactivated state 142–4, **142**, **143**, *144*
  and neurodivergence 244
  state identification 145, *145*
avoidance behaviours 38–9, 117–22, *119*, **120**
awe-seeking *262*

back injury 75
balance 44–7, 50–3, 55, 62, 165–6, 173, 254, 279, 286
  and activity 146–58
  biology balancing behaviour 133–66
  and symptom spirals 108
  tweaking activity for *150–1*, 154–8
  see also homeostasis; imbalance
basal ganglia 188, 199
Beck **111**
'behavioural experiments' 159–60, *161*
behaviours (responses)
  biology balancing 133–66
  destructive 124
  fixing 265
  safety increasing 158–62
  and symptom spirals 110, **111**, 112, 113–14, **116**
  which betray beliefs 291–5, *292–4*
being 155
being valued 15, 54, *284*
beliefs **199**, 200, 204, 216, *219*, 236, 272, 314–15

behaviours which betray 291–5,
292–4
causes/precipitators of 279–85
choosing new 295–7, *296*
conflicting 287
core 275–7, 279, 283, 290–1, *292*
developmental formation 280–3,
290
embodying new 297–9, *298*
for empowerment and safety
286–91
flexible 295
flipping 285
health 274–9, **276**, 283
threatening 283–5, *284*, **285**, 287,
290–5, *292–4*
updating 273–302
belonging, sense of 6, 168–9, 225,
227–8
binaries 281–2
binge-eating 62, 137, 188
biology **20**, 21, 30, 69, 69–70, 72, 271,
280, 304
balancing behaviour 133–66
befriending your 37–67
and emotions 169–73, **170**, 175–6,
178–9
and fatigue 81
and health 19
and pain avoidance 75
and sleep 79–80
and threat 309
working with your 99–101, 107
see also body; psychobiological
processes
biomedical model 96, 277–8, *296*
biometrics 135
bioplasticity 65–7, 69–70, 101, 117,
145, 162, 222, 241

Biopsychosocial Model 8–9, 12,
19–21, **20**, 31–2, **60**, 63, **64**, 69,
223, 277–8, 283, *296*, 327
black people 97, 238, 239
bladder issues ix–x, 6, 66, 89, 90–3,
99, 115, 201, 288
hyperactive 5, 92, 93
see also urinary tract infections
bladder pain syndrome 235–6
blanking out 124
blood sugar levels 43, 46, 62, 135, 141
bodily sensations 110, **111**, 112,
113–14, 115, **116**, 206, 235
body 327
balancing 44–7, 50–3, 55, 62,
107–8, 134, 136, 173, 228, 232,
244, 254, 279, 286, 319
befriending your 37–67, 99–101, 107
and bioplasticity 65–7, 69–70, 241
and the brain 47–9, **48**, 278–9
capacity for change 65–7, 69–70
cultivating safety in 5, 23, 29, 123
and dealing with criticism 252–3
development 280
dysregulation 62, 80, 84–7, 92, 124,
146, 162, 174–5
and emotions 169–73, **170**, 175–6,
178–9
feeling anger towards your 8,
99–100
and feeling unsafe 115, 117, 173–4,
204
hating your 38, 99–100
interconnectivity **48**, 278
messages of the 61–3, 75, 244, 326
recognising where it is at 141–5
regulation 14, 19, 38, 175
and sleep 137–9
and symptom spirals 110, 115, 117

body – *cont.*
  threatened 47–9, **48**, 65, 101, 107, 173–4, 198–201, 204, 210–11, 285, **285**, 287
  and trust issues 168–9, 191–2, 326, 327
  understanding your 12, 33–101
  see also biology; *mind–body...*
body clock (circadian rhythms) 79, 139, 140
Body Mind Connect 9
body positive experiences 155–6
bone marrow 83
bottom up processes **48**, 280, 298
bowel issues 9–11, 95, 109, 118, 152
  see also specific conditions
bowel movements 87
brain 5, 10, 13–16, 21–2, 32, 44–6, 89, 97, 134–5, 265–6, 304
  and aging 241–2
  and attention 198–9
  and automatic responses **170**, 172
  and 'being' 155
  and beliefs 279–83, 286–7, 295–9
  and the bladder 91–3, 92
  and blanking out 124
  and the body 47–9, **48**, 278–9
  and body positive experiences 156
  and busyness 57
  and cognitive dissonance 287
  and cognitive immunization 287–9
  and compassion 259–60
  connectivity 207
  and decentring 257–8
  development 54–5, 280–3
  and distraction 187–9
  dorsal (thinking) 119–20, 171–2, 175, 207
  and emotions 57, 169–73, **170**, 179–80, 183, 187–9
  and fatigue 80
  glutamate build-up within 77
  and headache/migraine 76
  hypersensitivity to bodily signals 235
  and imagery 220
  and inflammation 82
  and interoceptive awareness 107, 145
  and magic fixes 61
  making changes in your 36
  and mind-over-matter narratives 201
  and mindfulness 207
  and multidimensionality 314
  and neural networks 186
  and neuroplasticity 241
  and pain 72–6, **72**, 94–5
  and physical exercise 241–2
  and the regulatory systems 180
  reward system 71, 188, 255, 282
  rewiring the 295
  and safety 16, 82, 120–1, 280
  and self-defective narratives 232
  shortcuts of the **170**, 172, 183–6
  and sleep 78, 138, 139
  and social experience 226, 227–9, 231, 245, 250, 258
  structure 207
  and symptom spirals 110, 115, 119–21
  and thought 195–9, **196**, 202, 207, 216
  and threat 16, 22, 38, 41, 47–9, **48**, 54, 65, 71, 101, 120–1, 127, 129, 159, 162, 165, 190, 258, 283–6, 309–10

and trauma 49–50
and the triggering phase 59
and uncertainty 299
ventral (emotional) 120, 171, 207, 252
see also gut–brain axis; *specific anatomical regions of the brain*
brain fog 82–3, 174, 184, 226, 305
brain imaging 80, 82, 124, 163, 207, 211, 241–2, 259
brain injury 162–3
brain-spamming thoughts 126–9, *128*
brainwaves 197–8, *197*, 199–200, 259
breast cancer 189–90
breathing techniques 181–2
British Medical Journal, The 239
burnout ix–x, xi, 13, 17, 21, 31, 58, 66–7, 115, 318
   beliefs about 200
   and brain-spamming 127
   and compassion fatigue 258, 259
   and the mind–body connection 28
   and symptom spirals 117
   and values 311, 316
busyness 56–7, 149–50, 290

calcitonin gene-related peptide 76
cancer ix–x, 97, 189–90, 207
capabilities, increasing *27*
car accidents 220
cardiovascular system 46, 47, 77, 134, 135, 229
central sensitization 75
cerebellum 241
certainty 263
see also uncertainty
challenge 51–2
change 12, 35–6, 56, 65–7, 269–327
cherry-picking 287, 288–9

child development 280–1
   critical periods 280
childhood experience 54–5, 280
   and the onset of illness 53, 54–5, **60**, 63, 66, **276**
   and symptom spirals **113**
childhood illnesses 55
choice 134
   see also decision-making
chronic fatigue syndrome (CFS) 78, 80–2, 122, 246
   see also myalgic encephalomyelitis
climate change 228
cognitive behavioural therapy (CBT) 6, 10, 109, **111**, 125, 126, 204
cognitive deconstruction 231–2
cognitive defusion 211
cognitive dissonance 287
cognitive immunization 287–9
cognitive load 201, 241–2
cognitive processing (thinking) 20–1, 82, 105, 120, 127, *128*, 184, **213**, 241–2, 244, 244–5, 280–1, 282, 319
   see also thoughts
collective action *262*
comfort compromise 139
comfort zone 159–60, *161*
community, sense of 225, 268, 305, 321
   see also tribe, finding your
compassion 186, 205–7, 258–61, 271
compassion fatigue 258
compassion-focussed therapy 280
concentration difficulties 82–3
confidence *28*
conflict 19
conscious 107, 127, 289
   see also subconscious; unconscious

control, sense of 15, 17, 69, 105, 115, 232–45, *284*
coping, through busyness 56–7
coping phase 11, 308, **309**
cortisol 43, 47, 84, 93, 152
courage 31
Covid-19 pandemic 10, 56, 81, 244–5, 261
creativity 313
crisis phase 11, 308, 309, **309**
criticism, dealing with 252–3
cross organ sensitization 93
curiosity 205, 206, 310, 325
cystitis 1, 3
cytokines 226–7

Dana, Deb 190
dancing 241
decision-making 77, 78, 82
    see also choice
default mode network (DMN) 71, 155, 187–8
defences, subconscious 231–2, 286–7
depression 5, 70–2, 79, 109, 115, 189–90, 208, 218, 282, 313, 318, 324–5
despair 4, 6, 100, 168, 273, 286, 318, 325–6
diabetes 141, 239
diet 6, 87, 135, 154
digestion 87–8, 152
disability x, 21, 305–6
disconnection 14, 37, 58, 107, 124–5, 167–8, 231, 257, 316
distraction techniques 182, 186–9, *215*
distress 129, 149, 179, 182, 188, 202, 208, 231, 259, 300
doing 155, 156–8

dopamine 15, 71, 94, 188, 199
dopaminergic systems 57, 282
dysregulation 50–3, 188, 229
    see also body, dysregulation; emotional dysregulation

eating windows 154
elderly people 239–45
electrical impulses 195, **196**, 197–8, *197*, 199–200
embodiment practices 5
emotion identification spectrum 176, **176**
emotion regulation 14, 49, 174, 177, 188–91, 203, 207, 236–7
    'window of tolerance' 179, **180**, 181–2
    see also emotional dysregulation
emotional avoidance 188
emotional awareness 173–7, 179
emotional discomfort, reduction *27–8*
emotional dysregulation 22, 124, 175
emotional expression 189–90
emotional overidentification 125–6, 177
emotional processing 174
emotional reactivity 244
emotional reasoning 126, *128*, 171–2, 177, 288–9
emotional support 255, **256**
emotional suppression 124–5, 177, 179–80, 236–7, 248, 320
emotions 13, 20–1, 206
    acceptance 182–3
    adjusting the volume on 179–82, **180**
    automatic responses to **170**
    befriending 169
    benign 122–6

biological basis 169–73, **170**, 175–6, 178–9
and brain-spamming 127–8
and cognitive defusion 211
disconnecting from 124–5
and evolutionary theory 172
feeling calmly 181–2
and feeling yourself better 167–92
and the gut 88–90
making them safer 173–5, 179, 184, 187
meeting your 124
negative/difficult 57, 73–4, 122, 124, 169, 182, 187–8, 190, 231, 288
resistance to 124, 183–6
spotting and labelling 177–9, **178**
and symptom spirals 110, **111**, 112, **113–14**, **116**, 119–20, 122–6
and thoughts 204
unfixable 185, 191
your relationship with your 177–9, **178**
see also specific emotions
empathy 207
empathy fatigue 258–9
empowerment 19, 23–4, **24**, 29, 32, 38, 107, 117, 134, 169, 232, 286–91, 318
endings 320–1
endometrial pain 115
endometriosis ix–x, 94, 210, 234
endorphins 77, 94
engagement *27*
engulfment 305–6
enjoyment, shared 255
epigenetics 54, 81
ethnic minorities 237–9
evolutionary theory 15, 86, 117, 172, 226, 231, 266

expectations, health 217–18, *219*, *292*, 325
expressive writing 189–90
Eye Movement Desensitization and Reprocessing (EMDR) 13, 187, 220

fairness, sense of 15, *284*
fatigue 78, 80–2, 109, 121, 143, 146, 152, 159–60, *161*, 184, 189, 207–8, 218
fear 4, 82, 113, 115, 123, 124, 168, 172, 201, 312–13
fear-avoidance cycles 120, **120**
'feelings wheel' tool 177–9, **178**
fibromyalgia 62, 207
fight or flight (or freeze response) 41, 75, 92, 252
see also stress response, quick-fire (acute)
financial insecurity 228, 229
fixing behaviours 265
focus 323
follicular phase 94
fortune telling 127–8, *128*, 204
Freud, Sigmund 234

gender stereotypes 235–7, 246
genes 54, 79
genetics 54, 79, 81, 227
'getting better' 303–27
glutamate 77
goals *see* healing goals
grief 168, 182, 191, 225, 321
guilt 171, 172, 183, 315
gut contractions (peristalsis) 88
gut issues 6, 86–90, 112, 122, 174
see also bowel issues; *specific conditions*

gut microbiome 88–9, 97–8, 124, 135
gut–brain axis 89

habits
  attentional 162–5
  mental 203–4, *205*
  micro-habits 323
  retraining worry 213–16, **213**
  unhealthy 137
hair 96–9
happiness 258–9
Harris, Russ 309
headaches 72–4, 76–7, 95, 184, 227, 234
healing 267–8
  barriers to 1
  definitions of 22–3
  and feeling yourself better 167–92
  as non-linear process 6
  and thinking 193–223
healing goals 21–9, 30, 32, 274
  and balance 146
  mapping the chapters of 322
  and micro-habits 323
  motivating 23–6
  outcome (big-picture) goals 24–6, *27–8*, 29, 321–2
  prioritization 323
  process (stepping-stone) goals 24–6, *27–8*, 29, 321–2
  reflecting on 323–4
  reviewing 321–2
  setting 21–2, 24, 26–9, *27–8*, 322
healing journey
  adaptation phase 308–9, **309**
  coping phase 11, 308, **309**
  crisis phase 11, 308, 309, **309**
healing journeys 30–1, 271, 304–5, 307–9, **307**, **309**, 325, 326–7

health inequalities 239
health journeys 63, **64**, 65
health psychologists x, 1, 35
healthcare system experiences 229–30
  collaborative 278
heart attack 41, 229, 234
heart health 15, 229
heartfulness 206
helplessness 96, 313
  learned 54
hippocampus 20, 49, 50, 188, **196**, 241
Hippocrates 234
Hirsch **213**
homeostasis (balance) 45, 51, 62, 79–80, 134, 136, 173, 228, 232, 244, 286, 319
hope 23–4, 29–30, 32, 59, 99, 308, 320
hopelessness 5, 25, 237
hormonal fluctuations 95
hormonal replacement therapy (HRT) 96
hormones 91–3
  sex 47
  stress 42–3, 45–6, 84, 93, 142, 152–3, 203
  see also specific hormones
hospital recovery spaces 227–8
hostility 74, 238
hunger 61–2
hydration 135–6, 154
hyperarousal **180**, 181
hyperfocus 113
hypervigilance 15, 76, 146, 162, 163, 197, 201, 235
hypnotic suggestion 74–5
hypoarousal 179, **180**
hypothalamic-pituitary-adrenal (HPA) axis 42–3, 49, 71, 84, 92–3, 229

hypothalamus 16, 41, 47, 92, 220
hysteria 234

identity, loss of 306–9
illness 174
  acceptance 306
  balancing 306
  chronic x, 28, 117, 141, 175, 265, 271
  coexistence of the self and 305–9, **307, 309**
  commonalities of xi
  and the mind–body connection 28
  onset 53–9, **60**, 63, 66, **113, 276**
  over-responsibility for 14, 38, 166, 232–3, 322
  perceptions of **276**, 279
  and post-traumatic growth 318
  pushing your body through 58
  terminal 21–2, 305
  traumatic nature 13
  you are not your illness 305–6
  see also specific illnesses
imagery 24–5, *215*, 220–1
imbalance 50–1
immobilization injury 25
immune system 15, 46, 47, 62, 65, 83–6, 174, 189
  components 83–4
  and emotional suppression 124
  and fatigue 81, 82
  and imagery 220
  and the skin 97, 98
  and social experience 226–7, 229
  supporting 134, 135, 137
immunity, adaptive 84
individualism 230, 240, 261
inequality 15
infections 84–6
infertility 21

inflammation 15, 46, 220
  brain 82
  chronic 62
  and dysregulation 84–5
  and fatigue 82
  and migraine 76
  and a sense of purpose 313
  and the skin 97
  and social experience 227
  and symptom spirals 109
inflammatory bowel disease (IBD) 7, 62, 85, 87, 118, 207
informational support **256**
injury 75, 162–3
inner voice/dialogue 31, 280–1
inner-critic 257
insomnia 78–9
intellectualizing 125
intention 24, 25–6, 257, 295, 299, 323
'intention-behaviour gap' 165–6
interconnectivity **48**, 223, 225–6, 261, 278
internal family systems therapy (IFS) 183–7, 290
internalization 235, 236, 243–4, 283
interoceptive awareness 61–3, 76, 107, 134, 141, 143–6, **143**, *145*, 173–7, 179, 201, 206–7, 235, 244
irritable bowel syndrome (IBS) ix–x, 7, 10, 59, 89, 118, 207, 248
isolation 13, 14, 55, 58, 67, 186
'it's all in your head' 1–32, **17, 18**, 38, 70, 74, 101, 193, 277

job stress 172–3
justice, sense of 15, *284*

Kabat-Zinn, Jon 193, 205–6, 209, 211
karma 277

labels 281–2
letter-writing, to yourself 324, 326–7
limbic system 78, 120–1, 187
listening skills 265
longevity 311
loved ones 263–6, **267**
luteal phase 94, 95
lymph nodes 83
lymphatic system 83

magic fixes 59–61, 135
manifestation 26
marginalisation 233
maternity care 239
meaning 6, 16, 22, *284*, 295
medial prefrontal cortex (mPFC) 186
medical misogyny 234–5
medical trauma 229–30, 303–4
meditation, mindfulness 210
Mediterranean diet 135
memory 82–3, 203
   long-term 13
   'touchstone' 13, 63
   traumatic 50
men 235–7
menopause 96
menstrual cycle 94
   see also periods
mental health 7–9, **9**, 17, 19
   see also specific conditions
mental state 221–3
mental stimulation 136–7
metabolic dysfunction 81–2
metabolic system 46, 47, 134, 229
metacognitive awareness 203, 204, 289
microaggressions 238
middle ground 105

middle occipital gyrus 242
migraine 2–3, 5, 72–4, 76–7, 99–100, 115, 193–4, 210, 268
mind 8, 23, 107–8, 186, 327
   see also conscious; subconscious; unconscious
mind reading 127–8, *128*
mind–body communication x, 7, 8, 35, 106
mind–body connection 5, 7, 8, 12, 28, 35, 38, 47, 66, 101, 123, 271
   see also psychobiological processes
mind–body disharmony 124
mind–body interaction 8, 21, 31–2, 69–101
mind–body research 10, 12, 109
mind-over-matter narratives 200–3
mindful-self compassion (MSC) 205
mindfulness 5–6, 133, 162, 193–4, 205–16, 221–2, 228, 273
mindfulness-based cognitive therapy (MBCT) 205, 207
mindfulness-based stress reduction (MBSR) 205, 207, 209
mindset, fixed/growth 295, *296*
'mini-interrupters' 147–9, 155–6, *157*
mirror neurons 227
misogyny, medical 234–5
mistrust 13–14, 69, 168, 229, 326
mitochondria 81–2
mood difficulties/issues ix, 21, 30–1, 59, 69–70, 201
   and bad periods 94
   and doing 158
   and nervous system pacing diaries 149
   and sickness behaviour 86
   and sleep loss 79, 80
   and stress 141

morning routines 140
movement 136
  see also physical activity
Moyers, Bill 209
multidimensionality 61, 146, 299–302, **301**, 314–16, 320
multiple diagnosis ix–x, 35
multiple sclerosis 6, 7, 85, 141, 173, 174, 207–8, 312–13
multisensory integration 107, 122–3, 146, 206–7, 235, 244, 280
muscle, deconditioning 75–6
myalgic encephalomyelitis (ME) 78
  see also chronic fatigue syndrome

naps 139–40
National Health Service (NHS) 7, 9, 108–9, 209, 234, 236, 324–5
needs 307
  basic 15, 229, *284*
  core *284*
  safety 15–16, **17**, 50, 54, 229, 283, 291
  social **267**
nerves 72–3, 75, 77, 92–3, 97
nervous system 5, 15, 47, **48**, 65, 99, 174–5, 179, 181, 229–30
  and balance 146–58, 165–6
  barometer 141, **142**, 143, 147, 179, 181, 190, 323
  central 45
  dysregulation 44–5, 63, 82
  and emotions 124
  enteric 89
  and fatigue 80
  and inflammation 82
  and neurodivergence 244
  parasympathetic 44, 84, 92, 141–2, **142**, 152, 182
  peripheral 45
  recalibration 155–6
  regulation 40
  sympathetic 42, 57, 84, 92, 113, 141, 142, **142**, 229
  and thinking 201–3
  and threat 120, 190
  see also autonomic nervous system
nervous system pacing diary 147–54, **148**, *150–1*, 158
nervous system profiles 149–54
  boom/busters 154
  head-firsters 149–50, 153, 154
  observers 152–3
neural networks 186, 274–5, 283
neural pathways 41, 77, 82–3, 91, 109, 126, 188, 202, 220, 255, 274–5, 280, 282, 286, 315
neurobiology 283
neurodivergence 177, 242–5
  see also attention deficit hyperactivity disorder; autism
neuroendocrine system 45–6, 47, 134, 137, 229
neurons (nerve cells) 77, 92–3, **196**, 199, 202, 227, 274–5, 299
neuroplasticity 65, 162, 241
neuroscience 71, 119–20, 186–7, 198, 213–16, 222, 231, 241, 258–9, 282–3, 301
neurotransmitters 71, 76–7, 94–5, 140, **196**, 199
neurotrophins 93
Ngangkari healers 22
no, learning to say 248–50
nocebos 217–18, *219*, 277
nociception **72**, 73
non-judgement 205
noradrenaline (norepinephrine) 42, 43

Ochs, Nola 242
oestrogen 94–5
openness 105, 236–7, 310, 325
optimism 320
'otherness' 168
over-achievers 289–90
over-responsibility 14, 38, 166, 232–3, 322
overwhelm 39, 40, 309, 319
ovulation 94
oxytocin 222, 255, 282

pacing 133, 134, 146
   see also nervous system pacing diary
pain ix, 3, 5–6, 72–7, 85, 174, 184, 220, 267
   avoidance 75–6
   and the brain 72–6, **72**, 94–5
   and brain-spamming 128
   chronic 75, 108, 141, 185–6, 207, 246
   emotional (secondary) 74, 75
   gut-related 88
   layers of 74–5
   and magic fixes 59
   and mindfulness 207, 208
   and nervous system profiles 152
   pelvic 90–3
   period 94–5, 96
   perpetuation 75–6
   primary physical 74–5
   and safety behaviours 122
   sensitivity to 75–6, 86, 95
   and sleep 79
   and social experience 230
   and symptom spirals 109, 113, 122
pain alleviation 21, 74–5, 96, 218
pain behaviours 75–6
pain equation 72–3, **72**

panic 3, 115
panic attacks 41, 234
panic disorder 41, 122
parasympathetic nervous system (PNS) 44, 84, 92, 141–2, **142**, 152, 182
parietal cortex 199
participation, shared 255
passivity *247*, 248, 252
pelvic floor muscles 91, 93
pelvic problems 90–3
perfectionism 28–9
periods (menstruation) 46–7, 94–6
'permission to come back' *215*
personal growth, post-traumatic 317–20
physical activity 96, 121, 136, 241–2
physical health 7–9, **9**, 13, 17, **18**, 19, 22, **70**
pink noise 139
placebos 217–18, *219*, 277
pleasure 70–1, 155–6, 255
polycystic ovary syndrome (PCOS) 94
Polyvagal Theory 45, 257–8, 280
Porges, Stephen 257–8
positivity 126, 320
   toxic 320
post-exertional malaise 121
post-traumatic growth 317–20
post-traumatic stress disorder (PTSD) 49–50, 109, 188
postcentral gyrus 242
Power Threat Meaning Framework 14
powerlessness 15, 19, 29, 50, 60, 183, 188, 216, 232, 267, 277, 286, 310
practical support **256**
practitioner-patient power dynamic 278
pre-birth experience 53–5, **60**, **113**

prefrontal cortex (PFC) 49, 61, 78, 83, 91–2, 110, 117, 129, 162, 187, **196**, 198, 201, 203, 216, 220, 236–7, 259
pregnancy 234
present moment, being in the *214*
prioritization 323
problem-solving 281
progesterone 94–5
progress, celebration 26–7
prosocial behaviour *262*
prostaglandins 95
psoriasis 99
psychobiological loops 77, 85, 101, 257
  and the bladder 93
  and fatigue 82
  and gut issues 87
  and interoceptive awareness 175
  and pain 75, 76
  and periods 96
  and somatosensory amplification 97–8
  and symptom spirals 107, 131
psychobiological processes 8, 19–20, **20**, 57, 69–71, **70**, 75–6, 81, 134
  and beliefs 274–5
  and stress 232
  and symptom spirals 112, 113, **113**, 119
  and thoughts 195–200, *196*, **196**, **199**
  see also mind–body...
psychology 6, 13, 19, **20**, 21, 30, 69, 70, 72, 117
psychotherapy 8, **9**, 21, 109
  see also specific forms of psychotherapy
purpose 6, 16, 22, 311, 313
pushing down 124–5

racial/ethnic background 237–9
racism 97, 238–9
rationalization 287
reflective practice 323–4
reframing 287
regulatory systems 45–7, **48**, 50–2, 54–5, 58, 62–3, 65, 86, 165–6, 174, 180, 188
  and expressive writing 189
  and neurodivergence 244
  and pain 74
  and social safety 228
  support for 134–7, 145
  see also cardiovascular system; immune system; metabolic system; neuroendocrine system
reinforcement, positive 188, 282
relationships 14–15, 137
religion *262*
resistance, emotional 124, 183–6
rest 142, 152, 154
'rest and digest' mode 92
rheumatoid arthritis 62, 85
Ricard, Matthieu 258–9
risk-taking 236
rumination 71, 163, 207, 222, 281, 291, 313
run-up period 53, 55–8, **60**, 63, 66, **113**, **276**
running 77

sadness 49, 53, 74–5, 106, 123–4, 175, 182, 186, 281, 288
'safe spaces' 220, 221
safety 13–17, 21, 23, 29, **48**, 50, 53–4, 82, 107, 123, 134, 165, 172, 194–5, 206, 216, 280, 283–91, 313
  and beliefs 283–91

safety – *cont.*
   and emotions 172, 173–5, 179, 184, 187, 295
   middle ground to 19–21
   pillars of 14
   social 226–9, 231–3, 245–8, 267, 268, 280
   see also threat
safety behaviours 117–22, *118–19*, 158–62, 289
safety needs 15–16, **17**, 50, 54, 229, 283, 291
SAM system 42, 43, 49
savouring 190–1, 211, 263
sedentary lifestyles 95
self 123, 231
   authentic 313
   coexistence with illness 305–9, **307, 309**
   decentring 257–8, 300–1
   finding yourself 309–13
   loss of 306–9
   multidimensional nature 299–302, **301**, 314–16
   and works in progress 303–27
self-advocacy 246–8
self-blame 69, 98, 130, 168–9, 173, 195, 202
self-care 86, 315
self-compassion 206–7
self-connection *28*
self-criticism *128*, 203, 216
self-expression 189–90
self-focus 163, 257–8
self-growth 314–15, 367
self-harm 137
self-hate 4, 99–100, 231
self-realization 12, 269–327
self-subjugation 246, 251

self-therapy 323–4
self-transcendence 261–2, *262*
self-trust 13–14, 16, 62–3, 145, 146, 168–9, 191–2, 327
self-worth 2, 15, 216, 283, 314
sensory information 279–80
serotonin 76–7, 94
sexual intercourse, painful 91
shame 2, 90–1, 183, 235, 236
sickness behaviours 85–6, 96, 117
Siegel, Dan 179
significant others 263–6, **267**
silence 57–8
Singh, Fauja 242
situations, and symptom spirals 110, **111**, 112, **114**, **116**, 130
skin issues 96–9
sleep 52, 77, 78–81, 136
   architecting 137–40
   and the gut 88
   interrupted 78–9
   rapid eye movement (REM) 138, *138*
   stages of 137, *138*
sleep aids 139
sleep debt 79–80, 137–8
sleep deprivation 78–9, 138–9
sleep homeostasis 79–80
sleep pressure 79–80, 140
sleep times 140
sleep/wake cycles 154
smoking 236
social anxiety 56, 58, 165, 257
social barometers 226–8, 245, 266
social connection 19, 50–1, 86, 137, 146, 225, 232–3, 246, 254–61, 267–8, **267**, 305–6, 315, 319, 321
   see also disconnection
social exclusion 55, 74, 226, 228, 230–2, 238

social experience 19, **20**, 21, 69, 74, 137, 165, 167–8, 222–3, 225–68, 271
social needs **267**
social roles, valued 15
social safety 226–9, 231–3, 245–8, 267, 268, 280
social support 96, 230, 254, 255, **256**, 319
social threats 226–32, 234–5, 237–9, 245, 254, 257–8, 266
social withdrawal 79, 86, *119*, 232, 259
somatosensory amplification 97–8
spinal cord 45
spirituality *262*
spleen 84
stereotypes, gender 235–7, 246
stigma xi, 8, 81, 90, 97, 209, 233, 243–4, 265, 277
stress 21, 37–48, 51–3, 52, 56, 65
   as action 39, 40
   and alexithymia 177
   as automatic response 39
   avoidance 38–9
   balancing 44–7
   biology of 41
   and the bladder 93
   control over 39
   counterbalance 44
   healthy 52
   micromanagement 40–50
   normalized high levels of 56
   and physical health 19, 37–8
   and situational factors 130
   and sleep 79
   and somatosensory amplification 97–8
   as a stressor 38, 39
   and tension 91
   threat of 39–42, 51

   see also allostatic load (chronic stress)
stress hormones 42–3, 45–6, 84, 93, 142, 152–3, 203
   see also adrenaline; cortisol
stress management 13, 38, 205, 207, 209
stress response 15, 39, 40–8, 92, 164, 199
   and emotions 179
   quick-fire (acute) 41–4, 117, 141–2, 201
   sustained (chronic) 15, 41–5, 65, 84, 141, 201
stroke rehabilitation 141
stuck, being 136–7, 141, 286
subconscious 61–2, 76, 107, 119, 187, 245
   defences 231–2, 286–7
suffering 15, 30, 108, 168, 191, 204, 206–9, 232, 234–5, 246, 250, 258–9, 263, 265, 303–4, 309, 326
sugary foods 95, 137
suicide 5, 236–7, 261
supplements 6, 10
survival 231, 258, 283, 307
sympathetic nervous system (SNS) 42, 57, 84, 92, 113, 141, 142, **142**, 229
sympathetic-adreno-medullary (SMS) system 41
symptom spirals **111**, **113**, **114**, **116**, 134, 137, 138–9, 146, 194, 274, 282, 291, 306, 308
   interruption 107–31
symptoms
   remission *27*, 304
   transforming your experience of 12, 103–268
synapses **196**, 241, 274, 280

tension 76–7, 91, 174, 176, 181, 265, 303
terminal illness 21–2, 305
tests, 'normal' results 13
'tethering' 182
thalamus 199
therapy 2–6, 8, **9**, 12, 21, 57, 109
   end of 321
   time-limited 324–5
   see also specific forms of therapy
thought control 202
thought suppression 202
thought-logging 204, *205*, 289
thoughts 82, 105, 120, 127, *128*, 184, **213**, 241–2, 244, 244–5, 280–1, 282, 319
   all-or-nothing (categorical) 105, 127, *128*, 244, 282
   and attention 198–9, **199**
   automatic 129, 204, 216
   brain-spamming 126–9, *128*
   and cognitive defusion 211
   fortune telling 127–8, *128*, 204
   intrusive 129, 202–3
   letting go of 211–12, *214*
   and mental habits 203–4, *205*
   negative 126, 202–3, 204
   positive 126
   psychobiology of 195–200, *196*, **196**, **199**
   'sticky' 213–16
   and symptom spirals 110, **111**, 112, **113–14**, **116**
   thinking yourself better/sick 193–223
   your relationship with your 210–12, **213**
threat 14–16, 22, 38, 47–9, **48**, 59, 153, 156, 163, 168, 172, 179, 199, 200–1, 220, 308, 318, 325
   acknowledgement and awareness of past 54
   anticipation of 16
   and being unheard 58
   and the body 47–9, **48**, 65, 101, 107, 173–4, 198–201, 204, 210–11, 285, **285**, 287
   and the brain 16, 22, 38, 41, 47–9, **48**, 54, 65, 71, 101, 120–1, 127, 129, 159, 162, 165, 190, 258, 283–6, 309–10
   childhood 55
   of illness 13
   and safety behaviours 117, 158
   social 226–32, 234–5, 237–9, 245, 254, 257–8, 266
   of stress 39–42, 51
   and symptom spirals 115
   and thinking 202, 203
threat mode 16, 23, 29, 61, 65, 101, 107, 113, 120, 127, 135, 145–6, 158, 162, 169, 174–5, 195, 198, 206–7, 210–11, 283–7, 291, 309
threatening beliefs 283–5, *284*, **285**, 287, 290–5, *292–4*
tiredness 78, 80
tone 252–3
top down processes **48**, 280, 297–8
transcendence 261–3, *262*
trauma xi, 21, 65, 67, 174, 220, 257–8
   and alexithymia 177
   and the brain 49–50
   and distraction 188
   medical 229–30
   and mind–body connection 28
   and nervous system dysregulation 45
   and symptom spirals 117

and threatening beliefs 285
trauma-processing therapy 13, 187, 190, 220
  see also Eye Movement Desensitization and Reprocessing
tribe, finding your 254–7
  see also community, sense of
trigger traps 265–6
triggering phase 53, 58–9, **60**, 66, **113**, **276**
trust 229
  establishing after dysregulation 50–3
  see also mistrust; self-trust

uncertainty, toleration 289, 299
unconscious, making conscious 289
unheard, feeling 57–8, 253, 267
unwell, three phases of becoming 53–9, **60**, 63, 66, **276**
  pre-birth experience 53–5, **60**, **113**
  run-up period 53, 55–8, **60**, 63, 66, **113**, **276**
  triggering phase 53, 58–9, **60**, 66, **276**
urethra 92
urinary tract infections (UTIs) 92
  recurrent 1–6, 37–8, 63, 66, 112–15, **114**, **116**, 133, 159, 166–9, 179–80, 193–4, 208–9, 211, 225, 303–4, 314, 325
urination 92
urine, colour/smell 135–6
'use it or lose it' 242

vagina 90, 91
vagus nerve 40, 44
valued, being 15, 54, *284*
valued action 319
values 310–11, *312*, 314–16, *317*, 319
visceral hypersensitivity 89
vision 24
visualization 24–6, 220
vulnerability 31, 115, 117–18, 123, 156, 183, 216, 230–1, 236–7, 246, 250, 300, 317, 327

wake times 140, 154
wants 250–1
Western medical system 22, 37, 166
Willcox, Gloria 177
wins, celebrating small 26
womb, 'wandering' 234
worry 82, 97–8, 113, 163, 197, 203, 281, 291
  retraining habits 213–16, **213**, *214–15*
  types *214–15*
worthlessness 2, 15
wound healing 62, 84–5
writing, expressive 189–90

Link to Notes

All of the Endnote references for this book are available online. You can access them by scanning the QR code below.